This book is dedicated to the following midlevel providers in appreciation for their successful efforts to improve diabetes outcomes in the patients under their care:

Katherine Arce, NP; Wanda Butts, NP; Susan Campos, NP; Diana Cano, PA; Maria Blanco-Castellanos, RN; Antoinette Chavez, RN; Lenore Coleman, PharmD; Mary Rose Deraco, RN; Tamara Douglas, RN; Cynthia Dunlop, RN; Simi Gandhi, NP; Joyce Ivy, NP; Guy Keppler, NP; Lisa Kirchen, RN; Gina Lau, PharmD; Teresa Luna, RN; Nilda Molina, Pharm D; Maria Navar, NP; Mary Pearce, NP; Levi Ramos, NP; Beverly Rockwell, RN; Manuela Romo, RN; Carol Rosenburg, RN; Elizabeth Spinella, NP; Thelma Staples, NP; Christine Turner, PA; Alana Wilson, RN; Barbara Wisehart, NP; and any others whom I might have inadvertently missed.

Contents

Preface

The American Diabetes Association (ADA) has recommended a number of evidence-based guidelines that result in good diabetes outcomes (Table 1). It is important, however, to differentiate between process measures (e.g., number of appropriate tests ordered or examinations carried out per period of time or whether an indicated treatment is given) and outcome measures (e.g., actual results of the test or effect of treatment). Many attempts to improve diabetes care result in improved process measures. However, many studies also show that improved process measures often do not translate into improved outcome measures. Three outcome measures are particularly important for influencing diabetes complications: A1C, LDL cholesterol, and blood pressure levels. Unfortunately, only 2–13% of patients meet the goals of all three of these outcome measures (1–9).

A major reason why so few patients meet the goals of the outcome measures is that our current medical care system makes it difficult to make timely and appropriate clinical decisions (10). One way around this barrier is to give midlevel providers prescriptive authority when they follow approved detailed treatment algorithms under the supervision of a physician. When this is allowed to happen, A1C levels fall threefold more in patients under the care of these midlevel providers compared with usual care (11). I have been caring for people with diabetes in this manner for 25 years. My recent experience has been in a community clinic with a dedicated nurse caring for 545 low-income, minority diabetic patients. Using this approach resulted in a fall in A1C levels from 9.6 to 7.1%, with 56% meeting the ADA A1C goal, 92% meeting the ADA LDL cholesterol goal, 90% meeting the ADA systolic blood pressure goal, and 95% meeting the ADA diastolic blood pressure goal in patients followed for 9–12 months (12,13). Remarkably, 47% of the patients met all three ADA outcome goals compared with 2–13% in nine other published studies (1–9). In a larger inner-city hospital-associated outpatient department with the same population, 44% met the ADA A1C goal, 77% the LDL cholesterol goal, and 83% both the systolic and diastolic blood pressure goal. A total of 31% met all three. Patients had to have initial

Table 1. ADA Standards of Care

Guideline	Frequency	Goal
1. A1C	Every 6 months if goal attained; Every 3 months if greater	<7.0%
2. LDL cholesterol	Yearly or more often as necessary	<100 mg/dl[a]
3. Triglycerides	Yearly or more often as necessary	<150 mg/dl
4. Renal profile	Yearly or more often as necessary	
a) Dipstick for proteinuria: if ≥1+[b], ACE inhibitor unless contraindicated; if negative or trace, evaluation for microalbuminuria		
b) Microalbuminuria: if positive[c] and confirmed, ACE inhibitor unless contraindicated		
5. Blood pressure	Measured at every routine diabetes visit	<130/80 mmHg
6. Eye examination	Yearly dilated funduscopic exam, except in type 1 diabetic patients, who should receive one within 3–5 years of diagnosis	
7. Foot examination	Annual comprehensive foot examination (patients with neuropathy should have a visual inspection of their feet at every visit)	
8. Aspirin	75–162 mg/day unless contraindicated	
9. Smoking cessation		

[a]<70 mg/dl if patient has clinical evidence of CVD: if either goal cannot be reached, a 30–40% reduction from baseline is an acceptable alternative. [b]With infection and menstrual bleeding ruled out. [c]Either albumin-to-creatinine ratio >30 µg/mg or albumin concentration >20 mg/l.

A1C levels >8.0% before being accepted into this diabetes program, which routinely follows over 1,000 patients.

The purpose of this book is to provide a background for the treatment algorithms for glycemia, dyslipidemia, and hypertension and describe their use. Based on 25 years of experience (12–17) plus the published experience of others (11), I have no doubt that if these algorithms are followed, glycemic, lipid, and blood pressure outcome measures will improve considerably in people with diabetes.

References

1. Saydeh SH, Fradkin J, Cowie CC: Poor control of risk factors for vascular disease among adults with previously diagnosed diabetes. *JAMA* 291:335–342, 2004

2. Grant RW, Buse JB, Meigs JB, for the University HealthSystem Consortium (UHC) Diabetes Benchmarking Project Team: Quality of diabetes care in U.S. academic medical centers. *Diabetes Care* 28:337–342, 2005

3. McFarlene SI, Jacober SJ, Winer N, Kaur J, Castro JP, Wui MA, Guwa A, Gizycki HV, Sowers J: Control of cardiovascular risk factors in patients with diabetes and hypertension at urban academic medical centers. *Diabetes Care* 25:718–723, 2002

4. Kemp TM, Barr ELM, Zimmet PZ, Cameron AJ, Welborn TA, Colagiuri S, Phillips P, Shaw JE, on behalf of the AusDiab Committee: Glucose, lipid, and blood pressure control in Australian adults with type 2 diabetes: the 1999–2000 AusDiab. *Diabetes Care* 28:1490–1492, 2005

5. Turchin A, Shubina M, Pendergrass ML: Relationship of physician volume with process measures and outcomes in diabetes. *Diabetes Care* 30:1442–1447, 2007

6. Varma S, Boyle LL, Varma MR, Piatt GA: Controlling the ABCs of diabetes in clinical practice: a community-based endocrinology practice experience. *Diab Res Clin Pract* 80:89–95, 2008

7. Peterson KA, Radosevich DM, O'Connor PJ, Nyman JA, Prineas RJ, Smith SA, Arneson TJ, Corbert VA, Weinhandl JC, Lange CJ, Hannan PJ: Improving diabetes care in practice: findings from the TRANSLATE trial. *Diabetes Care* 31:2238–2243, 2008

8. Cheung BMY, Ong KW, Cherny SS, Sham P-K, Tso AWK, Lam KSL: Diabetes prevalence and therapeutic target achievement in the United States, 1999 to 2006. *Am J Med* 122:443-453, 2009

9. Holbrook A, Thabane L, Keshavjee K, Dolovich L, Bernstein B, Chan D, Troyan S, Foster G, Gerstein H, for the COMPLETE II Investigators: Individualized electronic decision support and reminders to improve diabetes care in the community: COMPLETE II randomized trial. *CMAJ* 181:37–44, 2009

10. Davidson MB: How our current medical care system fails people with diabetes: lack of timely, appropriate clinical decisions. *Diabetes Care* 32:370–372, 2009

11. Davidson MB: The effectiveness of nurse- and pharmacist-directed care in diabetes disease management: a narrative review. *Curr Diabetes Rev* 3:280–286, 2007

12. Davidson MB, Castellanos M, Duran P, Karlan V: Effective diabetes care by a registered nurse following treatment algorithms in a minority population. *Am J Manag Care* 12:226–232, 2006

13. Blanco-Castellanos M, Duran P, Davidson MB: A carve in model of nurse-directed diabetes care is as effective as a carve out model: preliminary results. *Diabetes* 58 (Suppl. 1):A593, 2009

14. Legorreta AP, Peters AL, Ossorio C, Lopez RJ, Jatulis D, Davidson MB: Effect of a comprehensive nurse-managed diabetes program: an HMO study. *Am J Manag Care* 2:1024–1030, 1996

15. Peters AL, Davidson MB: Application of a diabetes managed care program: the feasibility of using nurses and a computer system to provide effective care. *Diabetes Care* 21:1037–1043, 1998

16. Davidson MB: Effect of nurse-directed diabetes care in a minority population. *Diabetes Care* 26:2281–2287, 2003

17. Davidson MB, Karlan VJ, Hair TL: Effect of a pharmacist-managed diabetes care program in a free medical clinic. *Am J Med Qual* 15:137–142, 2000

Acknowledgments

I wish to acknowledge two people who were instrumental (for different reasons) for my success with detailed treatment algorithms to improve diabetes care. Twenty-five years ago, Richard C. Ossorio, MD, the Medical Director of the Cedars-Sinai HMO, was able to curb the high cost of HIV disease by directing these patients to several infectious disease specialists who developed a protocol for their care. After this success, Dr. Ossorio approached me to develop a program for the care of diabetic patients, and nurse-directed care was born. Writing detailed treatment algorithms was one of the most challenging intellectual exercises I've undertaken. This is because there can be no "clinical judgments" contained in them; there has to be a specific instruction for the midlevel provider depending on specific individual circumstances (i.e., the dose of the medications in response to the laboratory or self-monitored blood glucose results, LDL cholesterol concentrations, or blood pressure). Only when the circumstances fall outside of the treatment algorithms should the supervisory physician be called. For greatest efficiency, this interaction needs to be minimal. Anne L. Peters, MD, my fellow at the time Dr. Ossorio approached me, has a marvelously logical mind and was extremely helpful in compiling the original and early renditions of the treatment algorithms. I am grateful to both of them for starting me on this 25-year quest to improve diabetes care.

Finally, I wish to thank Ken Babamoto, PharmD, for providing the list of antihypertensive medications listed in Chapter 5.

Chapter 1
Laying the Groundwork

BACKGROUND FOR EVIDENCE-BASED ADA GUIDELINES FOR STANDARDS OF DIABETES CARE

Diabetes mellitus has a profound effect on the health of our population. Diabetic retinopathy is the leading cause of blindness in people between 20 and 74 years of age (1). Diabetic nephropathy is the leading cause of patients undergoing dialysis for end-stage renal disease (2). Diabetic peripheral neuropathy is the underlying cause of non-traumatic lower-extremity amputations in diabetic patients (3). More than half of lower-extremity amputations occur in people with diabetes (4), who at the time these data were collected constituted only 4.5% of the population (5). The prevalence of coronary artery disease is twofold higher in men with diabetes and fourfold higher in women with diabetes, compared with appropriate nondiabetic control subjects (6). Strokes are two to three times more common in people with diabetes than in people without the disease (7). Peripheral arterial disease is also much more common in diabetic patients than in nondiabetic individuals (8).

Much of this devastation can be avoided. The microvascular complications of diabetes could be markedly reduced, if not eliminated, if near-euglycemia is maintained. Progression of early kidney disease to late-stage nephropathy can be forestalled by appropriate (non-glycemic) therapy. Although macrovascular disease cannot be entirely prevented, its effects can be sharply curtailed with appropriate treatment for lipids and blood pressure, smoking cessation, and ingestion of aspirin. Evidence for these important assertions will be briefly summarized.

GLYCEMIA

There have been five studies in over 2,000 type 1 (9–11) and type 2 (12,13) diabetic patients demonstrating that there is virtually no development or progression of retinopathy and nephropathy over 4–9 years if mean A1C levels are maintained at <7.0%. Figure 1 shows this relationship in type 1 diabetic patients enrolled in the well-known Diabetes Control and Complications Trial (DCCT). In two of these studies (9,12), an intervention that lowered glycemia resulted in much less microvascular complications, proving a causative relationship between near-euglycemia and these improved outcomes.

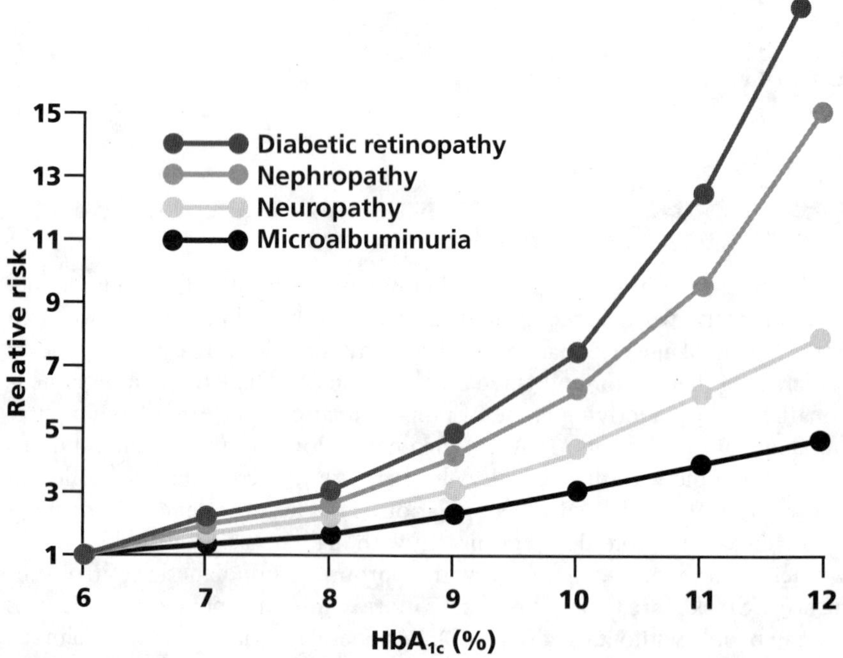

Figure 1. DCCT: Relative risk of progression of diabetic complications by mean HbA_{1c}.*

There is much less evidence that lowering glycemia will have a beneficial effect on macrovascular disease, at least in the near- to mid-term. Although there is an association between glycemia and cardiovascular disease (CVD), it extends all the way down into the mid-normal range (14). For instance, in men between the ages of 40 and 74 years, there was a 2.7-fold increase of a myocardial infarction in individuals with A1C levels between 5.0 and 5.4% compared with individuals with A1C levels <5.0% over 4 years (15). In another study involving nondiabetic adults, there was a 2.4-fold increase in the relative risk for a CVD event over 8–10 years for each 1% increase in A1C levels >4.6% (16).

In older individual studies (17) or in a meta-analysis (18), no beneficial effect was seen on CVD by lowering glycemia in type 2 diabetic patients. Three larger recent studies that focused specifically on the effect of glucose

---

***Based on DCCT data**

control on CVD also failed to demonstrate a beneficial effect. In the Action to Control Cardiovascular Risk in Diabetes (ACCORD) study (19), 10,251 patients (median baseline A1C level of 8.1%), 35% of whom had a previous CVD event, were randomized to receive intensive (goal A1C level of <6.0%) or usual care (goal A1C level of 7.0–7.9%). The study was stopped after 3.5 years because there was a significantly higher CVD mortality in the intensively treated group (achieved median A1C level of 6.4%) compared with the control group (achieved median A1C level of 7.5%) despite the fact that the intensively treated group had a significant reduction in nonfatal myocardial infarctions.

In the ADVANCE study (20), 11,140 patients (mean A1C level of 7.5%) with a history of major macrovascular or microvascular disease or at least one other risk factor for vascular disease (besides diabetes) were randomized to receive intensive glucose control (goal A1C ≤6.5%) or standard glucose control (targeted A1C defined on the basis of local guidelines). At the end of the study (median duration of 5 years), there was no difference in major macrovascular events (CVD death, nonfatal myocardial infarction, nonfatal stroke) between the intensively treated patients (achieved mean A1C of 6.5%) and the patients treated under standard conditions (achieved mean A1C of 7.3%). There was a significant reduction in the development of nephropathy in the intensively treated group, as has been found in many other studies evaluating microvascular complications.

In the Veterans Affairs Diabetes Trial (VADT) (21), 1,791 veterans (mean baseline A1C level of 9.4%) were randomized to receive intensive or standard treatment. A total of 40% of the cohort had had a prior CVD event. At the end of the study (median duration of 5.6 years), there was no difference in major CVD events (death, myocardial infarction, stroke, heart failure, amputation due to ischemia, intervention for coronary, or peripheral arterial disease) in the intensively treated (achieved A1C level of 6.9%) and standard (achieved A1C level of 8.4%) groups. As in the ADVANCE study, there was a significant decrease in the progression of albumin excretion in the intensively treated group.

Although there were no significant reductions in CVD events after a mean of 6.5 years of intensive treatment in type 1 diabetic patients, there was a significant decrease after a further 10.5 years (22). Similarly, in type 2 diabetic patients, there were no statistical differences in myocardial infarctions and death from any cause between intensive and conventional treatment after a median of 10.5 years, but significant reductions in both were seen in the intensively treated group after a further 10 years (23). These beneficial effects on macrovascular disease occurred despite the fact that between-group differences in A1C levels in both studies were lost within 1 year after the DCCT and U.K. Prospective Diabetes Study (UKPDS) were concluded, supporting the importance of near-euglycemia early in the course of diabetes.

Based on these data, the American Diabetes Association (ADA) recommends an A1C treatment goal of <7.0% (24), with which the author agrees.

LIPIDS

There is no doubt, of course, that lowering LDL cholesterol levels has a causative effect on reducing cardiac events in the general population (25). Lipid-lowering drugs are equally effective in reducing the relative risk of coronary disease in people with and without diabetes, i.e., the percent reduction is the same (26). However, the reduction of absolute risk is threefold greater in diabetic patients (26) because approximately three times as many people with diabetes are at risk for a CVD event than individuals without diabetes. Relative risk reduction is similar across all baseline LDL cholesterol levels (27) and is equally beneficial in older and younger diabetic patients (27,28) and in men and women (27). There is an ~20% relative risk reduction for a 40 mg/dl fall in LDL cholesterol levels (25,29). Not surprisingly then, cardiac events were 25% lower in diabetic patients receiving 80 mg atorvastatin compared with 10 mg (30). Treatment of ~30 type 2 diabetic patients with a statin will prevent one major cardiac event over 4 years (31,32). The use of statins has been shown to be cost-effective (33,34).

Based on these data, the ADA (24) recommends that all type 2 diabetic patients over the age of 40 years should receive a statin regardless of baseline LDL cholesterol levels. Statins should also be considered for younger patients at high risk for CVD. The goal for patients without clinical evidence of CVD is <100 mg/dl. For these with clinical evidence of CVD, the goal is <70 mg/dl.

What about triglyceride concentrations? Very high triglyceride levels (>1,000 mg/dl) can cause pancreatitis. Therefore, patients presenting with values >1,000 mg/dl should be treated initially with a fibrate. Because all diabetic patients >40 years of age will also be taking a statin, the fibrate should be fenofibrate, not gemfibrozil. The combination of a fibrate and a statin increases the risk of side effects. Fenofibrate is less likely to do so because it does not affect the pharmacokinetics of statins as gemfibrozil does.

Very few patients have high enough triglyceride levels to require initial fibrate treatment. Many patients, however, will have elevated triglyceride levels, and most of them have depressed HDL cholesterol levels. It is not clear whether the risk is mainly due to high triglyceride levels or low HDL cholesterol levels. Fenofibrate treatment of type 2 diabetic patients who were not taking a statin had much less of an effect on CVD (35) than published reports with statins. The National Cholesterol Education Program (36) and the ADA (24) suggest the following approach to triglyceride concentrations. Once the LDL cholesterol goal is reached, non-HDL cholesterol (total cholesterol minus HDL cholesterol) should be calculated in patients whose triglyceride levels are >200 mg/dl. Triglycerides are carried on many different lipoproteins, and non-HDL cholesterol levels reflect the more atherogenic ones. The goal for non-HDL cholesterol is <30 mg/dl above the LDL cholesterol goal.

RENAL EVALUATION

Many studies have evaluated the effects of either angiotensin-converting enzyme (ACE) inhibitors or angiotensin receptor blockers (ARBs) on renal disease in diabetic patients. Studies on patients with clinical proteinuria (i.e., albumin-to-creatinine ratios >300 µg/mg, 24-h urinary albumin >300 mg, 24-h urinary protein >500 mg), many of whom had renal insufficiency, used a primary end point of a doubling of serum creatinine levels and secondary end points of dialysis, renal transplant, or death. In randomized control trials, both an ACE inhibitor (37) and an ARB (38,39) significantly reduced these end points compared with a placebo. Either blood pressure levels were kept the same in the two groups (37) or the benefits were independent of blood pressure changes (38,39). Many smaller studies support these conclusions (40).

ACE inhibitors and ARBs also reduced the progression of microalbuminuria (30–300 µg albumin/mg creatinine) to clinical proteinuria (>300 µg/mg) and increased the return of microalbuminuria to normoalbuminuria (40). These effects were independent of changes in blood pressure. Studies in normotensive type 1 (41) and type 2 (42) diabetic patients, in which an ACE inhibitor significantly decreased the development of clinical proteinuria from microalbuminuria, prove this point. When the ACE inhibitor was discontinued (by patient choice), microalbuminuria returned (43), showing that the improvement was not due to natural variability. Finally, a meta-regression analysis showed that although blood pressure lowering decreased proteinuria and increased glomerular filtration rate, ACE inhibitors had an additional beneficial effect independent of its effect on blood pressure (44).

Based on these data, the ADA (24) recommends that, unless contraindicated, patients with microalbuminuria or clinical proteinuria be given either an ACE inhibitor or an ARB. Furthermore, one of these agents should be part of an anti-hypertension treatment regimen, again unless contraindicated.

HYPERTENSION

There is a difference in the patterns of hypertension between type 1 and type 2 diabetic patients. In the former, hypertension usually only occurs after patients develop renal disease. In the latter, hypertension is up to three times greater than in age- and gender-matched people without diabetes and is frequently present when type 2 diabetes is diagnosed. Lowering blood pressure in hypertensive individuals is certainly beneficial in the general population (45). What are the data in people with diabetes? Regarding CVD outcomes, three studies have compared intensive treatment of hypertension in diabetic patients with either placebo or usual care (46–48). Blood pressure levels, not surprisingly, were significantly lower in the intensively treated groups. In three other studies (49–51), diabetic patients were randomly assigned to different blood pressure targets, thus allowing an evaluation of different blood pressure levels on CVD events.

In the Hypertension Detection and Follow-up Program, patients were randomly assigned to intensive treatment versus referral to usual care (46). Subjects receiving intensive treatment had 38% less cardiovascular mortality and morbidity. In the Systolic Hypertension in the Elderly Program (SHEP), patients were also randomly assigned to intensive treatment or usual care by primary providers (47). On average, during the trial, the intensively treated diabetic patients had lower systolic and diastolic blood pressure levels of 9.8 and 2.2 mmHg, respectively, than the usual care group. There was a 34% reduction in total cardiovascular events and a 26% decrease in total mortality in the intensively treated group. In the Systolic Hypertension in Europe (Syst-Eur) study, patients were randomly assigned to nitrendipine or placebo (48). Systolic and diastolic blood pressure levels fell by 8.6 and 3.9 mmHg, respectively—more in the actively treated diabetic patients than in the placebo-treated group. There was a 70% reduction in cardiovascular mortality, a 65% reduction in all cardiovascular events, and, after adjustment for confounders, a 55% reduction in overall mortality in the patients receiving nitrendipine.

In the Hypertension Optimal Treatment (HOT) study, patients were randomly assigned to target diastolic blood pressures of 90, 85, or 80 mmHg (49). Achieved diastolic blood pressure levels were 85, 83, and 81 mmHg. The groups assigned to a diastolic blood pressure of 80 mmHg had a significant decrease in cardiovascular events of 51% and of total cardiovascular deaths of 44% compared with the group assigned to 90 mmHg. In the UKPDS, patients were randomized to a "tight" blood pressure group with a goal of <150/85 mmHg or a "less tight" blood pressure group of <180/105 mmHg (50). (The UKPDS was planned in the 1970s—thus, the high "less tight" goal.) The blood pressure levels actually achieved were 144/82 and 154/87 mmHg, respectively. There was a significant 34% reduction in total cardiovascular events and an 18% reduction in total mortality (the latter just missing significance) in the "tight" blood pressure group compared with the "less tight" group.

In the Appropriate Blood Pressure Control in Diabetes (ABCD) trial (51), patients were assigned to an intensive treatment group (target diastolic blood pressure of 75 mmHg) or a moderate control group (target diastolic blood pressure of 80–89 mmHg). Achieved blood pressure levels were 132/78 and

138/86 mmHg, respectively. Total mortality was significantly reduced by 49% in the intensively treated group compared with the moderate control group, but there was no difference in cardiovascular mortality to explain it.

Reducing blood pressure also reduced the risk for stroke. In the UKPDS (50), strokes were reduced by 44% in the "tight" control group compared with the "less tight" group. There was a 20% reduction in strokes in the SHEP study (47). The excess stroke risk associated with type 2 diabetes was abolished in the nitrendipine group in the Syst-Eur Study (48).

As noted above, it should be emphasized that the blood pressure control had a striking beneficial effect on the microvascular complications of diabetic patients as well (50,52). Furthermore, in patients with renal insufficiency, controlling blood pressure is the most important factor in preserving renal function (53). Based on these data, the ADA recommends a blood pressure goal of <130/80 mmHg (24). For patients with renal insufficiency, the National Kidney Foundation recommends an even lower blood pressure goal of <125/75 mmHg in patients with proteinuria exceeding 1 g/day (54).

Lowered blood pressure must be maintained to have a beneficial effect on the complications of diabetes. In the glycemic situation in the UKPDS, where despite the fact that A1C levels became similar in the intensively and conventionally treated groups soon after the active part of the study ended, a beneficial effect on both microvascular and macrovascular complications was seen over 10 years later. Differences in blood pressure between the two groups also disappeared within 2 years after the UKPDS ended, but the benefit of previously improved blood pressure was not sustained 10 years later (55).

EYE EXAMINATION

The main reasons for screening for diabetic retinopathy are that the process before visual loss is asymptomatic, and laser photocoagulation surgery, although effective in stabilizing vision, does not restore it. Two large randomized trials sponsored by the National Institutes of Health firmly established beneficial effects of this treatment for severe diabetic retinopathy (but not for mild or moderate disease). In the Diabetic Retinopathy Study (56), panretinal photocoagulation decreased the incidence of severe visual loss (best acuity of 5/200 or worse) by 50% during a 6-year follow-up, starting almost immediately.

The results of focal photocoagulation for macular edema (the most common retinal cause for visual loss in type 2 diabetic patients) in the Early Treatment Diabetic Retinopathy Study (57) were similar. The end point was a 50% deterioration in vision evaluated by an acuity chart (e.g., 20/40 to 20/80). After 3 years, 12% of the treated eyes compared with 24% of the untreated eyes had deteriorated to that extent. Further analysis revealed that only eyes with "clinically significant macular edema" needed to be treated because the rate of visual loss was very low in eyes with milder macular changes, and there was no evidence of benefit from treatment of this earlier process. Retinal thickening that occurs at or near the center of the macula is the hallmark of clinically significant macular edema. Unfortunately, this can only be assessed by stereo contact lens biomicroscopy and stereo photography, procedures not available to non-ophthalmologists (although exudates in the macular area almost always predict retinal thickening). To complicate matters further, initial visual acuity does not help select patients for further investigation. Even patients with normal visual acuity, but with clinically significant macular edema, were helped by focal macular photocoagulation. Thus, yearly eye examinations are extremely important for detecting macular edema that would benefit from laser photocoagulation surgery.

FOOT EXAMINATION

Eighty-five percent of lower-extremity amputations in diabetic patients are secondary to foot ulcers, most of which need not occur. Prevention of foot ulcers depends on identification of the early signs of foot pathology, areas of erythema and/or warmth, and calluses (which reflect increased pressure). It goes without saying that without examining the feet, one cannot identify early lesions, the treatment of which will prevent further damage and possible amputations.

ASPIRIN

A meta-analysis of 145 prospective controlled trials of antiplatelet therapy for secondary prevention of myocardial infarctions, strokes, or transient ischemic attacks revealed an ~25% reduction in recurrences in each of these outcomes (58). Diabetic patients had similar relative risk reductions but, as discussed above, they had higher absolute reductions in these events because of their increased risk for such events. Two randomized controlled studies of primary prevention that included diabetic patients also showed a beneficial effect of aspirin. The U.S. Physicians' Health Study (59) demonstrated a 44% reduction in myocardial infarctions in individuals receiving aspirin with a 61% reduction in the diabetic subgroup. In the HOT study (49), discussed above under "Hypertension," the diabetic hypertensive patients were also randomized to receive 75 mg aspirin or placebo. Aspirin significantly reduced cardiovascular events by 15% and myocardial infarctions by 36%. Finally, in the Early Treatment Diabetic Retinopathy Study (56), also discussed above under "Eye Examinations," the comparator group to photocoagulation was aspirin. Because ~10% of these patients had a history of CVD, this was a mixed primary and secondary prevention trial. The relative risk for myocardial infarction in the first 5 years of the study was lowered by 28% in individuals receiving aspirin (60).

The recent standards of care by the ADA (24) state that low-dose (75–162 mg/day) aspirin use for prevention is reasonable for adults with diabetes and no previous history of vascular disease who are at increased risk for CVD (10-year risk of CVD events over 10%) and who are not at increased risk for bleeding. Those adults with diabetes at increased CVD risk include most men over age 50 years and women over age 60 years, who have one or more of the following major risk factors: smoking, hypertension, dyslipidemia, family history of premature CVD, or albuminuria. Aspirin is not recommended for individuals at low CVD risk (women under 60 years of age and men under 50 years of age with no major CVD risk factors, who have a 10-year CVD risk under 5%), since the potential adverse effects from bleeding offset the potential benefits. Clinical judgment should be used for individuals who do not meet either of these criteria.

There was an ~60% increase in the relative risk of major gastrointestinal bleeding with aspirin (61). This is not reduced by enteric-coated aspirin. There is also a moderately increased risk in hemorrhagic stroke in patients taking aspirin, regardless of the dose. The absolute risk, however, is approximately one event per 1,000 users over 3–5 years. Aspirin does not increase retinal or vitreous hemorrhage (60).

Contraindications to aspirin use include allergy to aspirin, a bleeding tendency, anticoagulant therapy, recent gastrointestinal bleeding, history of a hemorrhagic stroke, and clinically active hepatitis. Because clopidogrel (Plavix) reduced CVD events in diabetic patients (62), it should be considered as alternative therapy for patients allergic to aspirin.

SMOKING CESSATION

A large body of evidence from a variety of studies (epidemiological, case-control, cohort) irrefutably documents the causal relationship between smoking and health risks (63). Smoking also increases the risk of microvascular complications in diabetic patients. Extensive public health efforts were associated with substantial reductions in smoking up to ~1990, after which about 25% of American adults, including people with diabetes, continued to smoke (64). Although certain forms of provider and behavioral counseling, as well as some drugs, have been clearly shown to reduce smoking, only about half of smokers with diabetes have been advised by their health care providers to quit smoking (63).

Based on these data, the ADA has recommended certain guidelines for diabetes care (24) that, if met, would markedly reduce the complications of diabetes (Table 2). When considering guidelines, it is important to distinguish between process measures and outcome measures. Process measures are the number of tests or examinations carried out per period of time or whether an indicated treatment is given. Outcome measures are the actual results of the test or the effect of the treatment. Unfortunately, simply meeting process measure goals often does not translate into improvement of outcome measures (65–67), e.g., frequent measurements of A1C levels do not necessarily lead to lowered glycemia.

RATIONALE FOR USING TREATMENT ALGORITHMS

Most diabetic patients do not meet the recommended goals in Table 2. Approximately half of the National Health and Nutrition Examination Survey (NHANES) cohort met the glycemic goal (68). In other reported populations, 21–43% of patients had A1C levels >9.5% (69–71). Only 22–46% of the general population of diabetic patients met the LDL cholesterol goal (72–75), and even in individuals with clinical evidence of CVD, only 60% had LDL cholesterols levels <100 mg/dl (75). Only 29–33% met the blood pressure goal (73,74) and, strikingly, 73% of diabetic patients had a blood pressure of >140/90 mmHg, a higher percentage than the 60% of nondiabetic patients (76). Far fewer (2–13%) met the combined ADA goals for the outcome measures of glycemia, lipids, and blood pressure (70,73,77–83). Many more studies have evaluated the process measures, and, sadly, carrying them out also remained far below the ADA guidelines (71,74,77,78,84–92). For example, fewer than half of diabetic patients take aspirin, ~75% of individuals with CVD but in only one-third of individuals without a history of myocardial infarction, angina, or a stroke (93), and only about half of smokers with diabetes have been advised by their health care providers to quit smoking (63).

An important barrier to good diabetes care is the lack of timely and appropriate treatment decisions. This is due to the lack of time that physicians have to spend with patients and not necessarily related to clinical inertia (see below). A primary care physician typically has 10–15 min with each patient. The vast majority of diabetic patients are asymptomatic, and their care involves prevention of the diabetic complications by controlling glycemia, lipid levels, and blood pressure and ensuring that the other process measures of diabetes care are carried out (Table 2). These issues often don't receive the attention they deserve, because other problems (especially those associated with symptoms) take priority. Moreover, patients are often seen only every 3 months or so, thus ensuring that glycemia, lipids, and blood pressure could remain out of control for long periods of time.

Table 2. Recommended ADA Treatment Guidelines

Guideline	Frequency	Goal
1. A1C	Every 6 months if goal attained; Every 3 months if greater	<7.0%
2. LDL cholesterol	Yearly or more often as necessary	<100 mg/dl[a]
3. Triglycerides	Yearly or more often as necessary	<150 mg/dl[b]
4. Renal profile	Yearly for albuminuria and every 6 months for serum creatinine or more often for each as necessary a) Dipstick for proteinuria: if ≥1+[c], ACE inhibitor unless contraindicated; if negative or trace, evaluation for microalbuminuria b) Microalbuminuria: if positive[d] and confirmed, ACE inhibitor unless contraindicated	
5. Blood pressure—Measured at every routine diabetes visit <130/80 mmHg		
6. Eye examination—Yearly dilated funduscopic exam, except in type 1 diabetic patients within 3–5 years of diagnosis; less frequent exams (every 2–3 years) may be considered in the setting of a normal eye exam; examination by retinal photographs (with or without pupil dilation) that are read by experienced experts can also be done.		
7.Foot examination—Annual comprehensive foot examination that should include assessment of protective sensation (with a Semmes-Weinstein 5.07 [10-g] monofilament), foot structure and biomechanics, vascular status, and skin integrity. Patients with neuropathy should have a visual inspection of their feet at every visit.		
8. Aspirin—75–162 mg/day for secondary prevention and in patients at increased risk[e] unless contraindicated		
9. Smoking cessation		

[a]<70 mg/dl if patient has clinical evidence of CVD: if either goal cannot be reached, a 30–40% reduction from baseline is an acceptable alternative. [b]See text for discussion of treating triglycerides; triglyceride goal is desirable but not an overt goal of pharmacotherapy. [c]With infection and menstrual bleeding ruled out. [d]Either albumin-to-creatinine ratio >30 µg/mg or albumin concentration >20 mg/l. [e]See text for discussion.

However, it is not just the long intervals of time between visits that account for the large proportion of diabetic patients who remain so far above the recommended goal levels for glycemia, lipids, and blood pressure. Clinical inertia—the lack of an appropriate treatment decision when the patient's clinical situation indicates that one should be made—is a major factor. For example, no change in therapy occurred within 90 or more days in diabetic patients taking oral antihyperglycemic medications whose A1C levels were >8.0% (94).

Diabetic patients treated with sulfonylurea agents had a mean of 4.5 A1C levels >8.0% before metformin was added on average 30 months later (95). The mean A1C levels when metformin was added to patients taking sulfonylurea agents, when sulfonylurea agents were added to patients taking metformin, and when insulin was started in patients taking the combination of the two oral medications were 9.6, 8.8, and 9.2%, respectively (96). Based on data from this large health maintenance organization in which A1C levels and medications were tracked over time, in the typical progression from nonpharmacologic therapy to monotherapy to combination therapy, patients spent nearly 5 years with A1C levels >8.0% and ~10 years with values >7.0% before starting insulin (96). In academic medical centers, only 40.4, 45.6, and 48.5% of diabetic patients had their medications changed with A1C levels >7.0, >8.0, or >9.0%, respectively (73). Only about one-half of patients failing a combination of metformin and a sulfonylurea with A1C levels >8.0% were started on insulin within 5 years (97). Only a slightly higher proportion were started with A1C levels >9.0% (97). In another study (98), physicians either added a new drug or increased the dose of an existing drug only ~20% of the time when A1C levels were >8.0%.

In the diabetic patients followed in the academic medical centers who were not taking a lipid medication, only 5.6, 8.7, and 15.4% had medication started with LDL cholesterol levels >100, >130, or >160 mg/dl (73). Similarly, in diabetic patients not treated for hypertension, only 10.1, 15.1, and 13.9% had an antihypertensive agent started with blood pressure levels >130/80, >140/90, or >150/100 mmHg, respectively (73).

Following the treatment algorithms for glycemia, lipid and blood pressure described in Chapters 3, 4, and 5 will ensure timely and appropriate clinical decisions and improve diabetes outcomes. For 25 years, I have trained and supervised nurses, pharmacists, and physician assistants to use these algorithms in caring for people with diabetes with gratifying results. For instance, in an especially challenging medically underserved minority population, a dedicated nurse following these algorithms in 545 patients for 9–12 months achieved a mean A1C level of 7.1%, with 57% meeting the ADA A1C goal of <7.0%, 87% meeting the LDL cholesterol goal of <100 mg/dl, 90% meeting the systolic blood pressure goal of <130 mmHg, and 95% meeting the diastolic blood pressure goal of >80 mmHg (99,100). If providers follow the treatment algorithms described in Chapters 3, 4, and 5, clinical inertia will be eliminated, timely and appropriate treatment decisions will be made, and patients will escape the potentially devastating complications of diabetes, or at least have them markedly attenuated.

References

1. Klein R, Klein BEK: Vision disorders in diabetes. In *Diabetes in America*. 2nd ed. National Diabetes Data Group, Eds. NIH publ. no. 95-1468, 1995, 293–338

2. Nelson RG, Knowler WC, Pettit DJ, Bennett PH: Kidney diseases in diabetes. In *Diabetes in America*. 2nd ed. National Diabetes Data Group, Eds. NIH publ. no. 95-1468, 1995, 349–400

3. Habershaw G: Foot lesions in patients with diabetes: cause, prevention, and treatment. In *Joslin's Diabetes Mellitus*. 13th ed. Kahn CR, Weir GC, Eds. 1994, 962–969

4. Reiber GE, Boyko EJ, Smith DG: Lower extremity foot ulcers and amputations in diabetes. In *Diabetes in America*. 2nd ed. National Diabetes Data Group, Eds. NIH publ. no. 95-1468, 1995, 409–428

5. Rubin RJ, Altman WM, Mendelson DN: Health care expenditures for people with diabetes mellitus, 1992. *J Clin Endocrinol Metab* 78:809A–809F, 1994

6. Wingard DL, Barrett-Connor E: Heart disease and diabetes. In *Diabetes in America*. 2nd ed. National Diabetes Data Group, Eds. NIH publ. no. 95-1468, 1995, 429–448

7. Kuller LH: Stroke and diabetes. In *Diabetes in America*. 2nd ed. National Diabetes Data Group, Eds. NIH publ. no. 95-1468, 1995, 449–456

8. Palumbo PJ, Melton LJ III: Peripheral vascular disease and diabetes. In *Diabetes in America*. 2nd ed. National Diabetes Data Group, Eds. NIH publ. no. 95-1468, 1995, 401–408

9. Skyler JS: Diabetic complications: the importance of control. *Endocrinol Metab Clin North Am* 25:243–254, 1996

10. Krolewski AS, Laffel LMB, Krolewski M, Krolewski M, Quinn M, Warram JH: Glycosylated hemoglobin and the risk of microalbuminuria in patients with insulin-dependent diabetes mellitus. *N Engl J Med* 332:1251–1255, 1995

11. Warram JH, Scott LJ, Hanna LS, Wantman M, Cohen SE, Laffel LMB, Ryan L, Krolewski AS: Progression of microalbuminuria to proteinuria in type 1 diabetes: nonlinear relationship with hyperglycemia. *Diabetes* 49:94–100, 2000

12. Ohkubo Y, Kishikawa H, Araki E, Miyata T, Isami S, Motoyoshi S, Kojima Y, Furuyoshi N, Shichiri M: Intensive insulin therapy prevents the progression of diabetic microvascular complications in Japanese patients with non insulin-dependent diabetes mellitus: a randomized prospective 6-year study. *Diabetes Res Clin Pract* 28:103–117, 1995

13. Tanaka Y, Atsumi Y, Matsuoka K, Onuma T, Tohjima T, Kawamori R: Role of glycemic control and blood pressure in the development and progression of nephropathy in elderly Japanese NIDDM patients. *Diabetes Care* 21:116–120, 1998

14. Barrett-Connor E, Wingard DL: "Normal" blood glucose and coronary risk: dose response effect seems consistent throughout the glycaemic continuum. *BMJ* 322:5–6, 2001

15. Khaw K-T, Wareham N, Luben R, Bingham S, Oakes S, Welch A, Day N: Glycated haemoglobin, diabetes, and mortality in men in Norfolk cohort of European prospective investigation of cancer and nutrition (EPIC-Norfolk). *BMJ* 322:15–18, 2001

16. Selvin E, Coresh J, Golden SH, Brancati FL, Folsom AR, Steffes MW: Glycemic control and coronary heart disease risk in persons with and without diabetes: the Atherosclerosis Risk in Communities Study. *Arch Intern Med* 165:1910–1916, 2005

17. Wild SH, Dunn CJ, McKeigue PM, Comte S: Glycemic control and cardiovascular disease in type 2 diabetes: a review. *Diabete Metab Res Rev* 15:197–204, 1999

18. Huang ES, Meigs JB, Singer DE: The effect of interventions to prevent cardiovascular disease in patients with type 2 diabetes. *Am J Med* 111:633–642, 2001

19. Action to Control Cardiovascular Risk in Diabetes Study Group: Effects of intensive glucose lowering in type 2 diabetes. *N Engl J Med* 358:2445–2559, 2008

20. ADVANCE Collaborative Group: Intensive blood glucose control and vascular outcomes in patients with type 2 diabetes. *N Engl J Med* 358:2560–2572, 2008

21. Duckworth W, Abraira C, Moritz T, Reda D, Emanuele N, Reaven PD, Zieve FJ, Marks J, Davis SN, Hayward R, Warren SR, Goldman S, McCarren M, Vitek ME, Henderson WG, Huang GD, for the VADT Investigators: Glucose control and vascular complications in veterans with type 2 diabetes. *N Engl J Med* 360:129–139, 2009

22. Diabetes Control and Complications Trial/Epidemiology of Diabetes Interventions and Complications (DCCT/EDIC) Study Research Group: Intensive diabetes treatment and cardiovascular disease in patients with type 1 diabetes. *N Engl J Med* 353:2643–2653, 2005

23. Holman RR, Paul SK, Bethel MA, Matthews DR, Neil HAW: 10 Year follow-up of intensive glucose control in type 2 diabetes. *N Engl J Med* 359:1577–1589, 2008

24. American Diabetes Association: Standards of medical care in diabetes–2010. *Diabetes Care* 33 (Suppl. 1):S11–S61, 2010

25. Cholesterol Treatment Trialist (CTT) Collaborators: Efficacy and safety of cholesterol-lowering treatment: prospective meta-analysis of data from 90 056 participants in 14 randomised trials of statins. *Lancet* 366:1267–1278, 2005

26. Costa J, Borges M, David C, Carneiro AV: Efficacy of lipid lowering drug treatment for diabetic and non-diabetic patients: meta-analysis of randomized controlled trials. *BMJ* 332:1115–1124, 2006

27. Wilt TJ, Bloomfield HE, MacDonald R, Nelson D, Rutks I, Ho M, Larsen G, McCall A, Pincros S, Sales A: Effectiveness of statin therapy in adults with coronary heart disease. *Arch Intern Med* 164:1427–1436, 2004

28. Neil HAW, DeMicco DA, Luo D, Betteridge DJ, Colhoun HM, Durrington PN, Livingstone SJ, Fuller JH, Hitman GA, on behalf of the CARDS Study Investigators: Analysis of efficacy and safety in patients aged 65-75 years at randomization: Collaborative Atorvastatin Diabetes Study (CARDS). *Diabetes Care* 29:2378–2384, 2006

29. Law MR, Wald NJ, Rudnicka AR: Quantifying effect of statins on low density lipoprotein cholesterol, ischaemic heart disease, and stroke: systematic review and meta-analysis. *BMJ* 326:1423–1429, 2003

30. Shepherd J, Barter P, Carmena R, Deedwania P, Fruchart J-C, Haffner S, Hsia J, Breazna S, LaRosa J, Grundy S, Waters D, for the Treating to New Targets Investigators: Effect of lowering LDL cholesterol substantially below currently recommended levels in patients with coronary heart disease and diabetes: the Treating to New Targets (TNT) study. *Diabetes Care* 29:1220–1226, 2006

31. Colhoun HM, Betteridge DJ, Dunnington PN, Hitman GA, Neil HAW, Livingtone SJ, Thomason MJ, Mackness MI, Menys VC, Fuller JH, on behalf of the CARDS Investigators: Primary prevention of cardiovascular disease with atorvastatin in type 2 diabetes in the Collaborative Atorvastain Diabetes Study (CARDS): multicentre randomized placebo-controlled trial. *Lancet* 364:685–696, 2004

32. Vijan S, Howard RA: Pharmacologic lipid-lowering therapy in type 2 diabetes: background paper for the American College of Physicians. *Ann Intern Med* 140:650–658, 2004

33. Brandle M, Davidson MB, Schriger DL, Lorber BL, Herman WH: Cost effectiveness of statin therapy for the primary prevention of major coronary events in individuals with type 2 diabetes. *Diabetes Care* 26:1796–1801, 2003

34. Heart Protection Study Collaborative Group: Lifetime cost effectiveness of simvastatin in a range of risk groups and age groups derived from a randomized trial of 20 536 people. *BMJ* 333:1145–1149, 2006

35. FIELD Study Investigators: Effects of long-term fenofibrate therapy on cardiovascular events in 9795 people with type 2 diabetes mellitus (the FIELD study): randomized controlled trial. *Lancet* 366:1849–1861, 2005

36. Grundy SM, Cleeman JI, Merz CNB, Brewer HB, Clark LT, Hunninghake DB, Pasternak RC, Smith SC, Stone NJ, for the Coordinating Committee of the National Cholesterol Education Program: Implications of recent clinical trials for the National Cholesterol Education Program Adult Treatment Panel III guidelines. *Circulation* 110:227–239, 2004

37. Lewis EJ, Hunsicker LG, Bain RP, Rohde RD, for The Collaborative Study Group: The effect of angiotensin-enzyme inhibition on diabetic nephropathy. *N Engl J Med* 329:1456–1462, 1993

38. Brenner BM, Cooper ME, de Zeeuw D, Keane WF, Mitch WE, Parving HH, Remuzzi G, Snapinn SM, Zang Z, Shahinfar S, for the RENAAL Study Investigators: Effects of losartan on renal and cardiovascular outcomes in patients with type 2 diabetes and nephropathy. *N Engl J Med* 345:861–869, 2001

39. Lewis EJ, Hunsicker LG, Clarke WR, Berl T, Pohl MA, Lewis JB, Ritz E, Atkins RC, Rhode BS, Ras I, for the Collaborative Study Group: Renoprotective effect of the angiotensin-receptor antagonist irbesartan in patients with nephropathy due to type 2 diabetes. *N Engl J Med* 345:851–860, 2001

40. Strippoli GFM, Craig M, Deeks JJ, Schena FP, Craig JC: Effects of angiotensin converting enzyme inhibitors and angiotensin II receptor antagonists on mortality and renal outcomes in diabetic nephropathy: a systematic review. *BMJ* 329:828–838, 2004

41. Laffel LMB, McGill JB, Grans DJ: The beneficial effect of angiotensin-converting enzyme inhibition with captopril on diabetic nephropathy in normotensive IDDM patients with microalbuminuria. *Am J Med* 99:497–504, 1995

42. Ravid M, Savin H, Jutrin I, Bental T, Katz B, Lishner M: Long-term stabilizing effect of angiotensin-converting enzyme inhibition on plasma creatinine and on proteinuria in normotensive type II diabetic patients. *Ann Intern Med* 118:577–581, 1993

43. Ravid M, Lang R, Rachmani R, Lishner M: Long-term renoprotective effect of angiotensin-converting enzyme inhibition in non-insulin-dependent diabetes mellitus. *Arch Intern Med* 156:286–289, 1996

44. Kasiske BL, Kalil RSN, Ma JZ, Liao M, Keane F: Effect of antihypertensive therapy on the kidney in patients with diabetes: a meta-regression analysis. *Ann Intern Med* 118:129–138, 1993

45. Chobanian AV, Bakris GL, Black HR, Cushman WC, Green LA, Izzo JL, Jones DW, Materson BJ, Oparil S, Wright JT, Roccella EJ: The seventh report of the Joint National Committee on Prevention, Detection, Evaluation, and Treatment of High Blood Pressure: the JNC Report. *JAMA* 289:2560–2572, 2003

46. Hypertension Detection and Follow-Up Cooperative Group: Five-year findings of the Hypertension Detection and Follow-Up Program. I. Reduction in mortality of persons with high blood pressure, including mild hypertension. *JAMA* 242:2562–2571, 1979

47. Curb JD, Pressel SL, Cutler JA, Savage PJ, Applegate WB, Black H, Camel G, Davis BR, Frost PH, Gonzales N, Guthrie G, Oberman A, Rutan GH, Stamler J. Effect of diuretic-based antihypertensive treatment on cardiovascular disease risk in older diabetic patients with isolated systolic hypertension: Systolic Hypertension in the Elderly Program Cooperative Research Group. *JAMA* 276:1886–1892, 1996

48. Tuomilehto J, Rastenyte D, Birkenhager WH, Thujs L, Antikanen R, Bulpitt CJ, Fletcher AE, Forette F, Goldhaber A, Palatini P, Sarti C, Fagard R, for the Systolic Hypertension in Europe Trial Investigators: Effects of calcium channel blockade in older patients with diabetes and systolic hypertension. *N Eng J Med* 340:677–684, 1999

49. Hansson L, Zanchetti A, Carruthers SG, Dahlof B, Elmfeldt D, Julius S, Menard J, Rahn KH, Wedel H, Westerling S, for the HOT Study Group: Effects of intensive blood-pressure lowering and low-dose aspirin on patients with hypertension: principal results of the Hypertension Optimal Treatment (HOT) randomized trial. *Lancet* 351:1755–1762, 1998

50. U.K. Prospective Diabetes Study Group: Tight blood pressure control and risk of macrovascular and microvascular complications in type 2 diabetes: UKPDS 38. *BMJ* 317:703–713, 199

51. Estacio RO, Jeffers BW, Hiatt WR, Biggerstaff HL, Gifford N, Schrier RW: The effect of nisoldipine as compared with enalapril on cardiovascular outcomes in patients with non-insulin-dependent diabetes and hypertension. *N Engl J Med* 338:645–652, 1998

52. Schrier RW, Estacio RO, Esler A, Mehler P: Effects of aggressive blood pressure control in normotensive type 2 diabetic patients on albuminuria, retinopathy and strokes. *Kidney Int* 61:1086–1097, 2002

53. Parving HH, Anderson AR, Smidt UM, Hommel E, Mathiesen ER, Svenden PA: Effect of antihypertensive treatment on kidney function in diabetic nephropathy. *BMJ* 294:1443–1447, 1987

54. Rossert JA, Wauters J-P: Recommendations for the screening and management of patients with chronic kidney disease. *Nephrol Dial Transplant* 17 (Suppl 1):19–28, 2002

55. Holman RR, Paul SK, Bethel MA, Neil HAW, Matthews DR: Long term follow-up after tight control in blood pressure in type 2 diabetes. *N Engl J Med* 359:1565–1576, 2008

56. Diabetic Retinopathy Study Group: Photocoagulation treatment of proliferative diabetic retinopathy: clinical application of diabetic retinopathy study (DRS) findings. DRS report number 8. *Ophthalmology* 88:583–600, 1981

57. Early Treatment Diabetic Retinopathy Study Research Group: Photocoagulation for diabetic macular edema; early treatment diabetic retinopathy study report number 1. *Arch Ophthalmol* 103:1796–1806, 1985

58. Antiplatelet Trialists' Collaboration: Collaborative meta-analysis of randomised trials of antiplatelet therapy for prevention of death, myocardial infarction, and stroke in high-risk patients. *BMJ* 324:71–86, 2002

59. Final report on the aspirin component of the ongoing Physicians' Health Study Research Group. *N Engl J Med* 321:129–135, 1989

60. ETDRS Investigators: Aspirin effects on mortality and morbidity in patients with diabetes mellitus: Early Treatment Diabetic Retinopathy Study report 14. *JAMA* 268:1292–1300, 1992

61. American Diabetes Association: Aspirin therapy in diabetes. *Diabetes Care* 27 (Suppl. 1):S72–S73, 2004

62. Bhatt DL, Marso SP, Hirsch AT, Ringleb PA, Hacke W, Topol EJ: Amplified benefit of clopidogrel versus aspirin in patients with diabetes mellitus. *Am J Cardiol* 90:625–628, 2002

63. Haire-Joshu D, Glasgow RE, Tibbs TL: Smoking and diabetes (Technical Report). *Diabetes Care* 22:1887–1898, 1999

64. American Diabetes Association: Smoking and diabetes. *Diabetes Care* 27 (Suppl. 1):S74–S75, 2004

65. McGinn J, Davis C: Geographic variation, physician characteristics, and diabetes care disparities in a metropolitan area. *Diab Res Clin Pract* 72:162–169, 2006

66. Ackermann RT, Thompson TJ, Selby JV Safford MM, Strevens M, Brown AF, Venkat Narayan KM: Is the number of documented diabetes

process-of-care indicators associated with cardiometabloic risk factor levels, patient satisfaction, or self-related quality of diabetes care? The Translating Research into Action for Diabetes (TRIAD) study. *Diabetes Care* 29:2108–2113, 2006

67. Mangione CM, Gerzoff RB, Williamson DF, Steers WN, Kerr EA, Brown AF, Waitzfelder BE, Marrero DG, Dudley RA, Kim C, Herman W, Thompson TJ, Safford MM, Seby JV, for the TRIAD Study Group: The association between quality of care and the intensity of diabetes disease management programs. *Ann Intern Med* 145:107–116, 2006

68. Hoerger TJ, Segel JE, Gregg EW, Saadine JB: Is glycemic control improving in U.S. adults? *Diabetes Care* 31:81–86, 2008

69. Davidson MB: The case for "outsourcing" diabetes care. *Diabetes Care* 26:1608–1612, 2003

70. Saydeh SH, Fradkin J, Cowie CC: Poor control of risk factors for vascular disease among adults with previously diagnosed diabetes. *JAMA* 291:335–342, 2004

71. Suwattee P, Lynch JC, Pendergrass ML: Quality of care for diabetic patients in a large urban public hospital. *Diabetes Care* 26:563–568, 2003

72. Jacobs MJ, Kleisli T, Malik S, L'Italien GJ, Chen RS, Wong ND: Prevalence and control of dyslipidemia among persons with diabetes in the United States. *Diab Res Clin Pract* 70:263–269, 2005

73. Grant RW, Buse JB, Meigs JB, for the University Healthsystem Consortium (UHC) Diabetes Benchmarking Project Team: Quality of diabetes care in U. S. academic medical centers. *Diabetes Care* 28:337–342, 2005

74. Beaton SJ, Nag SS, Gunter MJ, Gleeson JM, Sajjan SS, Alexander CM: Adequacy of glycemic, lipid, and blood pressure management of patients with diabetes in a managed care setting. *Diabetes Care* 27:694–869, 2004

75. Yan AT, Yan RT, Tan M, Hackam DG, Leblanc KL, Kertland H, Tsang JL, Jaffer S, Kates ML, Leiter LA, Fitchett DH, Langer A, Goodman SG, for the Vascular Protection (VP) and Guidelines Oriented Approach to Lipid Lowering (GOALL) Registries Investigators: Contemporary management of dyslipidemia in high-risk patients: targets still not met. *Am J Med* 119:676–683, 2006

76. Berelowitz DR, Ash AS, Hickey EC, Glickman M, Friedman R, Kader B: Hypertension management in patients with diabetes. *Diabetes Care* 26:355–359, 2003

77. McFarlene SI, Jacober SJ, Winer N, Kaur J, Castro JP, Wui MA, Gliwa A, von Gizycki H, Sowers JR: Control of cardiovascular risk factors in patients with diabetes and hypertension at urban academic medical centers. *Diabetes Care* 25:718–723, 2002

78. Kemp TM, Barr ELM, Zimmet PZ, Cameron AJ, Welborn TA, Colagiuri S, Phillips P, Shaw JE, on behalf of the AusDiab Steering Committee: Glucose, lipid, and blood pressure control in Australian adults with type 2 diabetes: the 1999–2000 AusDiab. *Diabetes Care* 28:1490–1492, 2005

79. Turchin A, Shubina M, Pendergrass ML: Relationship of physician volume with process measures and outcomes in diabetes. *Diabetes Care* 30:1442–1447, 2007

80. Varma S, Boyle LL, Varma MR, Piatt GA: Controlling the ABCs of diabetes in clinical practice: a community-based endocrinology practice experience. *Diab Res Clin Pract* 80:89–95, 2008

81. Peterson KA, Radosevich DM, O'Connor PJ, Nyman JA, Prineas RJ, Smith SA, Arneson TJ, Corbert VA, Weinhandl JC, Lange CJ, Hannan PJ: Improving diabetes care in practice: findings from the TRANSLATE trial. *Diabetes Care* 31:2238–2243, 2008

82. Cheung BMY, Ong KW, Cherny SS, Sham P-K, Tso AWK, Lam KSL: Diabetes prevalence and therapeutic target achievement in the United States, 1999 to 2006. *Am J Med* 122:443–453, 2009

83. Holbrook A, Thabane L, Keshavjee K, Dolovich L, Bernstein B, Chan D, Troyan S, Foster G, Gerstein H, for the COMPLETE II Investigators: Individualized electronic decision support and reminders to improve diabetes care in the community: COMPLETE II randomized trial. *CMAJ* 181:37–44, 2009

84. Saaddine JB, Engelgau MM, Beckles GL, Gregg EW, Thompson TJ, Venkat Narayan KM: A diabetes report card for the United States: quality of care in the 1990's. *Ann Intern Med* 136:565–574, 2002

85. Chin MH, Zhang HX, Merrell K: Diabetes in the African-American Medicare population: morbidity, quality of care, and resource utilization. *Diabetes Care* 21:1090–1095, 1998

86. Greenfield S, Kaplan SH, Kahn R, Ninomiya J, Griffith JL: Profiling care by different groups of physicians: effects of patient case-mix (bias) and physician-level clustering on quality assessment results. *Ann Intern Med* 136:111–121, 2002

87. Grant RW, Cagliero E, Murphy-Sheehy P, Singer DE, Nathan DM, Meigs JB: Comparison of hyperglycemia, hypertension, and hypercholesterolemia management in patients with type 2 diabetes. *Am J Med* 112:603–609, 2002

88. Acton KJ, Shields R, Rith-Najarian S, Tolbert B, Kelly J, Moore K, Valdez L, Skipper B, Gohdes D: Applying the diabetes quality improvement project indicators in the Indian Health Service primary care setting. *Diabetes Care* 24:22–26, 2001

89. Srinivasan M, Przyblski M, Swigonski N: The Oregon Health Plan: predictors of office-based diabetic quality of care. *Diabetes Care* 24:262–267, 2001

90. Porterfield DS, Kinsinger L: Quality of care for uninsured patients with diabetes in a rural area. *Diabetes Care* 25:319–323, 2002

91. Petitti DB, Contreras R, Ziel FH, Dudl J, Domurat ES, Hyatt JA: Evaluation of the effect of performance monitoring and feedback on care process, utilization, and outcome. *Diabetes Care* 23:192–196, 2000

92. Demakis JG, Beauchamp C, Cull WL, Denwood R, Eisen SA, Logren R, Nichol K, Woolliscraft WG, for the Department of Veterans Affairs Cooperative Study Group on Computer Reminders in Ambulatory Care: Improving residents' compliance with standards of ambulatory care: results from the VA Cooperative Study on Computerized Reminders. *JAMA* 284:1411–1416, 2000

93. Persell SD, Baker DW: Aspirin use among adults with diabetes: recent trends and emerging sex disparities. *Arch Intern Med* 164:2492–2499, 2004

94. Wetzler P, Snyder JW: Linking pharmacy and laboratory data to assess the appropriateness of care in patients with diabetes. *Diabetes Care* 23:1637–1641, 2000

95. Brown JB, Nichols GA: Slow response to loss of glycemic control in type 2 diabetes mellitus. *Am J Manag Care* 9:213–217, 2003

96. Brown JB, Nichols GA, Perry A: The burden of treatment failure in type 2 diabetes. *Diabetes Care* 27:1535–1540, 2004

97. Rubino A, McQuay LJ, Gought SC, Kvasz M, Tennis P: Delayed initiation of subcutaneous insulin therapy after failure of oral glucose-lowering agents in patients with type 2 diabetes: a population-based analysis in the UK. *Diabet Med* 24:1412–1418, 2007

98. Shah BR, Hux JE, Laupacis A, Zinman B, van Walraven C: Clinical inertia in response to inadequate glycemic control: do specialists differ from primary care physicians? *Diabetes Care* 28:600–606, 2005

99. Davidson MB, Castellanos M, Duran P, Karlan V: Effective diabetes care by a registered nurse following treatment algorithms in a minority population. *Am J Manag Care* 12:226–232, 2006

100. Davidson MB, Blanco-Castellanos M, Duran P, Verma M, Dayrit M, Somillon A, Naheed S, Akhanjee L: Effect of nurse-directed care for reducing disparities in diabetes outcomes: a carve in vs. a carve out model. *Diabetes* 57 (Suppl. 1):A339, 2008

Chapter 2
Evidence-Based Principles of Dietary Therapy

I have been involved in diabetes research, care, and teaching for over 40 years, and the literature during this period describing diet treatment of diabetes is one of the most controversial areas in diabetes. Most of the "principles" cannot be confirmed by subsequent studies, and no agreement backed by high levels of evidence has been reached about what is the best mix of calories (i.e., amounts and forms of carbohydrates, protein, and fat) for people with diabetes. In my view, only four aspects of dietary therapy that affect clinical outcomes have been firmly established:

1. Patients taking two or more injections of insulin per day in a mixed-split regimen should eat (and exercise) consistently each day. Mealtimes and carbohydrate content of each meal must be (relatively) consistent from day to day. Basal/bolus regimens allow more flexibility.
2. The more carbohydrate a meal contains (regardless of form), the greater the postprandial rise of glucose concentrations.
3. Dietary saturated and trans fats increase circulating total and low density lipoprotein (LDL) cholesterol concentrations.
4. Most importantly, overweight and obese patients require hypocaloric diets.

Most providers (certainly physicians) are not trained to give detailed instructions to patients concerning diet. This type of guidance should be given by a registered dietitian or a certified diabetes educator (CDE), who has received special training in dietary counseling. However, physicians should be able to determine the appropriate amount of calories that the patient requires and provide that to the person carrying out the nutritional counseling. (In my experience, if this is not done, often either no caloric level is given to the patient or the amount mentioned is often too high for significant weight loss.) Table 3 summarizes how to arrive at an appropriate caloric level (which also applies to diets for people without diabetes).

Table 3. Calculating the Caloric Content of (Diabetic) Diets

1. Desirable body weight (DBW)

a.	Females	Males
First 5 ft	100 lb	106 lb
Each inch over 5 ft	5 lb	6 lb

b. Frame Size: Ten percent is added to the DBW for large-framed individuals, and 10% is subtracted for small-framed subjects. Frame size can be estimated by having the patient's predominant hand grasp the other wrist and oppose the thumb and middle finger. If these two fingers meet, the patient has a medium frame (and no DBW adjustment is necessary). If they overlap appreciably, the patient is small framed. If they fail to meet, the patient is large framed. Appropriate adjustments are made to the DBW in the latter two circumstances. Patients who are ≥120% of DBW (i.e., ≥20% over their DBW) are considered overweight or obese, and patients <120% of DBW are considered lean.

2. Calorie content
   To lose weight: 10 calories per lb of DBW
   To maintain weight: 15 calories per lb of DBW
   To gain weight: 20 calories per lb of DBW
   Lower limit: 1,000 calories

3. Age
   <50 years: No change
   50–60 years: Subtract 10% from calorie content, if sedentary
   >60 years: Subtract 20% from calorie content, if sedentary
   Lower limit: 1,000 calories

An inconvenient fact is that 1 lb of fat contains ~3,500 calories (9 calories/g × 453.6 g/lb). Thus, to lose 1 lb of fat, a patient must be in a 3,500-calorie deficit (i.e., over whatever period of time a patient expends 3,500 more calories than is ingested, 1 lb of fat will be lost). The approach in Table 3 yields an ~500-calorie deficit per day, which should result in a 1-lb weight loss per week. If this diet were followed faithfully, the patient would safely lose ~50 lb per year.

An important caveat must be kept in mind. Fluid-wise, the body adjusts to the carbohydrate intake. A decrease in carbohydrate intake results in a diuresis. Because hypocaloric diets invariably contain less carbohydrate than patients usually consume, there is an initial diuresis, and more weight is lost than the decreased calories should yield in the first several weeks. The more obese the patient, the greater the initial weight loss due to diuresis. Much of the greater initial weight loss of low-carbohydrate, high-fat diets (e.g., Atkins diet) is due to the greater diuresis secondary to the very low intake of carbohydrates compared with a diet with similar calories but higher carbohydrate content. Conversely, if a dieting patient binges, the increased carbohydrate intake leads to fluid retention, and more weight is gained than can be attributed to the extra calories per se.

Unfortunately, the long-term response to hypocaloric diets is disappointing. Many patients (slightly over half) will initially lose some weight (up to 5-10% of initial weight) during the first 6 months or so, but regain of most of this weight is commonly seen in the maintenance phase (1–3). Exercise is important to the successful maintenance of weight loss (4,5). To make matters worse, there is some evidence that people with diabetes may have more difficulty losing weight and keeping it off (3,6,7). These disappointing results with diet and exercise as successful lifestyle interventions in newly diagnosed diabetes are a major reason why the American Diabetes Association recommends metformin treatment (along with diet and exercise) at the time of diagnosis (8).

Much controversy exists concerning the importance of the form of carbohydrates in the diet. A patient eating an apple has a modest rise in glucose concentrations. That same apple ingested as applesauce produces a greater increase. If the apple is made into apple juice, the increase is even greater than that seen with the applesauce. However, when different sources of carbohydrate are folded into a meal, the postprandial rise in glucose levels mostly depends on the total amount of carbohydrate, not its form. This even applies to such sources of carbohydrate as sucrose (table sugar).

Dietitians and CDEs specially trained in nutritional counseling will, no doubt, be disappointed by the brevity of this chapter. However, the criterion for discussing the principles of dietary therapy for people with diabetes is that these principles must be firmly established as evidence-based. The principles presented here meet that criterion and, in my view, other information concerning dietary therapy does not.

References

1. McTigue KM, Harris R, Hemphill B, Lux L, Sutton S, Bunton AJ, Lohr KN: Screening and interventions for obesity in adults: summary of the evidence for the U.S. Preventive Services Task Force. *Ann Intern Med* 139:933–949, 2003

2. Franz MJ, VanWormer JJ, Crain AL, Boucher JL, Caplan HT, Bowman JD, Pronk NP: Weight-loss outcomes: a systematic review and meta-analysis of weight-loss clinical trials with a minimum 1-year follow-up. *J Am Diet Assoc* 107:1755–1767, 2007

3. Dansinger ML, Tatsioni A, Woong JB, Chung M, Balk EM: Meta-analysis: the effect of dietary counseling for weight loss. *Ann Intern Med* 147:41–50, 2007

4. Svetsky LP, Stevens VJ, Brantley PJ, Appel LJ, Hollis JF, Loria CM, Vollmer WM, Gullion CM, Funk K, Smith P, Samuel-Hodge C, Myers V, Lien LF, Laferriere D, Kennedy B, Jerome GJ, Heinith F, Harsha DW, Evans, P, Erlinger TP, Dalcin AT, Coughlin J, Charleston J, Champagne CM, Bauck A, Ard JD, Aicher K, for the Weight Loss Maintenance Collaborative Research Group: Comparison of strategies for sustaining weight loss: the Weight Loss Maintenance Randomized Controlled Trial. *JAMA* 299:1139–1148, 2008

5. Jakicic JM, Marcus BH, Lang W, Janney C: Effect of exercise on 24-month weight loss maintenance in overweight women. *Arch Intern Med* 168:1550–1559, 2008

6. Pi-Sunyer FX: Weight loss in type 2 diabetic patients. *Diabetes Care* 28:1526–1527, 2005

7. Franz MJ: The dilemma of weight loss in diabetes. *Diabetes Spectrum* 20:133–135, 2007

8. Nathan DM, Buse JB, Davidson MB, Ferrannini E, Holman RR, Sherwin R, Zinman B: Medical management of hyperglycemia in type 2 diabetes: a consensus algorithm for the initiation and adjustment of therapy: a consensus statement of the American Diabetes Association and the European Association for the Study of Diabetes. *Diabetes Care* 32:193–203, 2009

Chapter 3
Glycemia

GOALS OF THERAPY

As discussed in Chapter 1, there is no longer any doubt that near-euglycemia will delay, and possibly prevent, the microvascular (retinopathy and nephropathy) and neuropathic complications of diabetes in both type 1 and type 2 diabetic patients. The American Diabetes Association (ADA) suggests the following goals for glycemic control: preprandial glucose, 70–130 mg/dl; postprandial glucose, <180 mg/dl; A1C level, <7.0%.

A1C value is referenced to a nondiabetic range of 4.0–6.0% in an assay standardized to the Diabetes Control and Complications Trial (DCCT)-based method. A level of <7% reflects near-euglycemia throughout the day and night and, if maintained from diagnosis, will prevent the development or progression of the microvascular complications of diabetes.

PRINCIPLES OF TREATMENT

Type 1 diabetic patients require insulin. Type 2 diabetes is a progressive disease; β-cell function continues to decrease regardless of which therapies are used. Therefore, although initial treatment with metformin (along with diet and exercise) is often successful, over time, more than one oral drug is required; eventually, insulin is necessary in the majority of type 2 diabetic patients. Although lifestyle modification (diet and exercise) is to be used initially and reinforced throughout therapy, metformin should be started at diagnosis for the following reasons: *1*) even if diet and exercise alone may be effective initially, it is difficult to sustain, and the vast majority of patients will soon require drug treatment; *2*) in the United Kingdom Prospective Diabetes Study (UKPDS), metformin was associated with less cardiovascular disease (CVD) (two-thirds of type 2 diabetic patients die from CVD); *3*) serious side effects to metformin are very rare; and *4*) metformin causes mild weight loss or at least weight stabilization.

There are four criteria to use when selecting a class of drugs or a drug within that class from among its competitors: *1*) effectiveness, *2*) side effects, *3*) ease of use (i.e., adherence to treatment), and *4*) cost. With the exception of insulin (the most effective if used appropriately), no drug or class of drugs stands out as much more effective than any others. A1C levels are used to judge the glycemic effect of drugs. It is extremely important to realize that the higher the initial A1C level, the greater the fall after an intervention. Thus, older drugs (sulfonylurea agents [SUs] and metformin), tested when glycemic control was worse than recently when newer drugs were evaluated, would seem more effective because the decreases in A1C levels were greater. However, when compared with the newer drugs at comparable A1C levels, this may not be the case.

A consensus conference was held by the ADA in the spring of 2008 to update their recommendations for the treatment of type 2 diabetes (1), which are depicted in Figure 2. When lifestyle plus metformin is no longer able to achieve

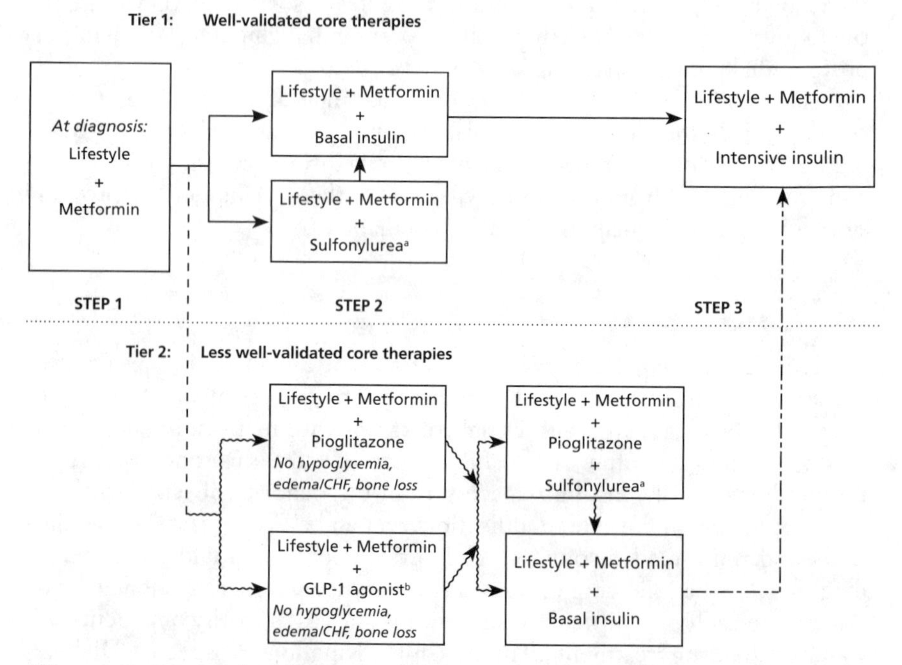

Figure 2. ADA's algorithm for the metabolic management of type 2 diabetes. Reinforce lifestyle interventions at every visit, and check A1C level every 3 months until <7.0%, and then measure at least every 6 months. The intervention should be changed if A1C is ≥7.0%. [a]Sulfonylureas other than glyburide or chlorpropamide. [b]Insufficient clinical use to be confident regarding safety. CHF, coronary heart failure. (Reprinted with permission from the American Diabetes Association.)

an A1C level <7.0%, the preferred route of therapy for most patients with type 2 diabetes is to add either an SU or basal insulin. An alternative (although not as enthusiastically recommended) is to add either pioglitazone or a glucagon-like peptide (GLP)-1 agonist. If either of these fail to achieve an A1C level <7.0%, metformin, pioglitazone, and an SU (triple oral therapy) could be considered, or basal insulin substituted for the GLP-1 agonist. In any event, if these approaches fail to achieve an A1C level of <7.0%, intensification of insulin should be the next step. The consensus conference did not recommend using glyburide or chlorpropamide, because of their increased potential to cause hypoglycemia compared with other SUs, or rosiglitazone, because of its possible deleterious effect on coronary artery disease compared with pioglitazone.

The use of metformin along with intensification of insulin therapy, i.e., two or more injections per day, is mainly to restrain weight gain. If insulin is used appropriately, the oral drug doesn't add much. Therefore, it should be discontinued in lean patients. Given the four criteria for drug selection described above, Figure 3 is a flow diagram of my general approach to treating type 2

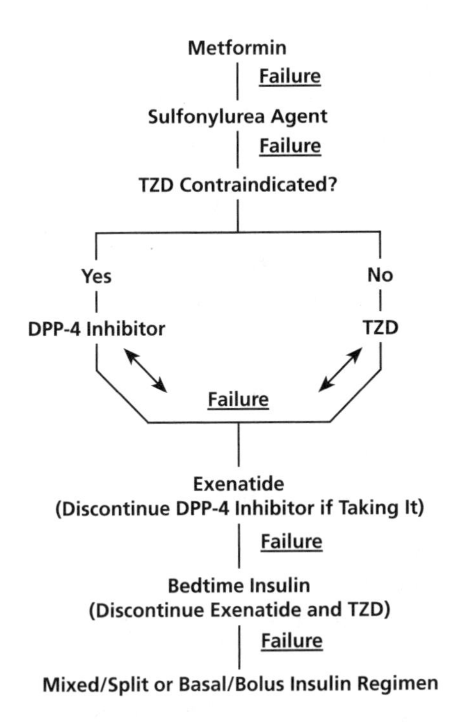

Figure 3. Flow diagram of the general approach to the treatment of type 2 diabetes.

diabetes, which is not inconsistent with the ADA recommendations. Dipeptidyl peptidase (DPP)-4 inhibitors were not recommended by the Expert Committee because their long-term safety had not been established. However, a recent publication found no difference in adverse events in 3,415 patients exposed to the DPP-4 inhibitor sitagliptin compared with 2,724 non-exposed patients followed for up to 2 years (2). Therefore, if pioglitazone is contraindicated, a DPP-4 inhibitor should be used before embarking on injection therapy. Although both SUs and DPP-4 inhibitors stimulate insulin secretion, they do it by different mechanisms. There is published evidence that adding sitagliptin to patients already on an SU will significantly lower A1C levels (3). Furthermore, patients failing a combination of maximal (tolerated) doses of metformin plus an SU respond similarly to the addition of a thiazolidinedione (TZD) or sitagliptin, at least acutely (4). Finally, in patients failing oral medications, adding exenatide or insulin glargine yields similar improvements in A1C levels (5,6). Insulin requires self-monitoring of blood glucose (SMBG) for dose adjustments and raises the possibility for hypoglycemia, neither of which is involved with exenatide.

Although each class of drugs will be discussed in more detail below, Table 4 summarizes their advantages and disadvantages.

The following explains the reasoning in Figure 3. The rationale for using metformin first has already been described. An SU is added to metformin failures because SUs are inexpensive, serious hypoglycemia is uncommon, and there is only mild weight gain. TZDs are effective in the majority of patients when added as a third oral drug (7) and are just as effective as bedtime NPH insulin when compared head-to-head in patients failing on metformin and an SU (8). The arguments for trying an oral incretin (a DPP-4 inhibitor) as the third drug in patients in whom a TZD is contraindicated follow: *1*) as already mentioned, sitagliptin was effective when added to metformin plus an SU (3) (despite the fact that the mechanism of action of both SUs and DPP-4 inhibitors is to stimulate insulin secretion, albeit by different mechanisms); *2*) if an oral incretin was not used in this situation, the next drug is an injectable one; and *3*) since the maximal effect on an easy parameter to follow (i.e., fasting plasma glucose [FPG] concentrations) is evident by 3 weeks, patients failing the DPP-4 inhibitor will be recognized quickly and transitioned to other therapy.

An injectable GLP-1 analog (exenatide) is not considered earlier in the treatment algorithm because of possible adherence to treatment issues (injection and its common side effect nausea) and cost. However, the common weight loss associated with it may make the GLP-1 analog attractive for some patients as a second-line drug. Insulin is reserved until last because of adherence to treatment issues. Besides requiring injections, insulin also requires SMBG and has the very real potential of hypoglycemia, as mentioned above. Bedtime insulin (plus pills) is the initial insulin regimen because it is often

Table 4. Comparison of the Classes of Drugs Used to Treat Glycemia in Type 2 Diabetes

Drug	Advantages	Disadvantages
Metformin	No hypoglycemia No weight gain; slight loss in some Oral administration	Adverse gastrointestinal effects common Slow dose titration Some contraindications (e.g., renal insufficiency, hepatic dysfunction, alcoholism, >80 years of age) Potential for lactic acidosis if used inappropriately Must be discontinued under certain circumstances and restarted Dosing usually twice (or three times) a day
SUs*	Effects seen quickly Few adverse effects Dosing often once a day Available as cheaper generics Oral administration	Hypoglycemia Some weight gain
TZDs (rosiglitazone, pioglitazone)	No hypoglycemia Dosing once daily Can be used in patients with renal failure Oral administration	Slow onset of effect Weight gain (fat accumulation) Edema (fluid retention) May precipitate heart failure, especially in patients also taking insulin Very expensive Decreased bone mineral density and increased fractures
Incretin analogs (exenatide)	Weight loss No hypoglycemia	Injected Initial nausea common Expensive
DPP-4 inhibitors (sitagliptin) (saxagliptin)	Weight neutral No hypoglycemia Oral administration	Expensive
α-Glucosidase inhibitors (acarbose, miglitol)	No hypoglycemia No weight gain	Flatulence common Very slow dose titration Dosing three times a day More expensive than metformin and sulfonylurea agents Contraindicated if creatinine ≥2 mg/dl Contraindicated in patients with intestinal disorders
Insulin	Most effective drug	Injected SMBG required Hypoglycemia Weight gain Consistency of lifestyle (eating and exercise) required

*Includes repaglinide (Prandin) and nateglinide (Starlix), non-sulfonylureas that are also insulin secretagogues acting on the same receptor as the SU compounds (but at a different site) in the pancreatic β-cell. Principles of use for repaglinide and nateglinide are the same as for SUs, except that they need to be given before each meal.

effective for long periods (9–12), only requires one injection and one SMBG test before breakfast, and does not usually put the patient at risk for daytime hypoglycemia. Two or more injections of insulin are used last because of the multiple injections, the requirement for more SMBG testing, the potential for daytime hypoglycemia, and the loss of flexibility in the patient's diet and exercise pattern (at least in patients using a mixed/split regimen).

Type 2 diabetic patients not taking insulin have a relatively stable FPG concentration (13,14). A provider can take advantage of this when starting or titrating doses of metformin and an SU, two drugs that have a strong effect on fasting glycemia and show it within 2–3 weeks. This aspect of type 2 diabetes is not as helpful for drugs that have their major effects on postprandial glucose concentrations (α-glucosidase inhibitors, glinides, GLP-1 analogs, DPP-4 inhibitors) or the TZDs with their delayed effect.

Two things must be stressed regarding the treatment protocol in Figure 3. First, formulary issues may affect the suggested treatments. Second, and very importantly, when a therapy has failed, the patient must be advanced to the next therapy quickly. The goal is to achieve near-euglycemia. However, there are five considerations to address before seeking near-euglycemia. These are *1*) limited life expectancy, *2*) the presence of advanced microvascular complications (tight control will have no effect at this point), *3*) severe CVD (tight control has little effect on CVD, and hypoglycemia can be detrimental), *4*) hypoglycemia unawareness (extremely uncommon in type 2 diabetic patients), and *5*) the inability or unwillingness to comply with the necessary regimen. In the absence of any of these, near-euglycemia (i.e., an A1C level of <7.0%) should be sought. In general, an A1C level of 6.0% corresponds to an average plasma glucose concentration throughout the day and night of 125 mg/dl, with an increase of ~30 mg/dl for each 1.0% increase in A1C levels (15).

NON-INSULIN DRUGS

METFORMIN

Mechanism of action. Metformin acts mainly by decreasing hepatic glucose production (probably by inhibiting gluconeogenesis). Some (but not all) studies show a more minor effect on increasing the ability of insulin to increase glucose utilization by muscle tissue, i.e., increasing insulin sensitivity or decreasing peripheral insulin resistance. Animal studies show that the drug may inhibit the absorption of glucose by the small intestine, although this has not been confirmed in humans. There is agreement that the drug does not increase insulin secretion.

Principles of use. Because of the common (usually temporary) gastrointestinal (GI) adverse effects that occur when metformin is started or the dose is increased, it is important to start with a small dose (500 twice daily) and increase it gradually. If the patient experiences GI adverse effects they will occur during the first week, usually with subsequent marked improvement or disappearance of these symptoms. (To minimize these symptoms, metformin should be taken with meals.) The FPG concentration should be measured 2–3 weeks after starting metformin and 2–3 weeks after each dose change. The short-term goal is to achieve a value of <130 mg/dl. If that goal is not achieved, and any GI symptoms that may be present are tolerable, the dose of metformin is increased by one step (see Incremental Step Doses and Maximal Final Doses below) until *1*) the FPG concentration becomes <130 mg/dl, *2*) the GI symptoms are intolerable (in which case, the dose should be reduced by one step), or *3*) the maximal dose is reached.

As long as the FPG concentration remains above 130 mg/dl, the dose of metformin should be increased by one step, and the FPG concentration measured in 2–3 weeks until the value falls below 130 mg/dl, at which time the dose is maintained and FPG and A1C levels are measured 3 months later. If the A1C level is <7.0% at that time (regardless of the FPG concentration), the dose of metformin is maintained, and both tests should be repeated every 3 months. On the other hand, if the A1C level is ≥7.0%, the dose of metformin is increased by one step (or if already at the maximal dose, an initial dose of an SU is added; see Sulfonylurea Agents and Glinides below). The protocol for assessing a dose increase is then followed (i.e., measuring the FPG concentration in 2–3 weeks if it was ≥130 mg/dl). It is unnecessary to repeat the FPG concentration in 2–3 weeks if the target has been met (i.e., <130 mg/dl) and the dose increase or the addition of an SU occurred because the A1C was ≥7.0. In that case, the FPG and A1C levels should be repeated in 3 months, and the evaluation process described in this paragraph followed.

Whenever intolerable GI symptoms to metformin occur, the dose should be reduced by one step, and the patient re-evaluated. This will usually occur after a dose increase, which implies that satisfactory control had not yet been achieved before the increase. In this case, combination oral therapy should be strongly considered. If, on the other hand, intolerable GI symptoms occur after the patient has been on a stable dose of metformin, an A1C level should be measured 3 months after the one-step decrease in dose. If the value is <7.0%, the dose is maintained, and the patient evaluated with A1C levels every 3 months. If the value is ≥7.0%, combination oral therapy with an SU should be started.

If the maximal dose of metformin is reached, and the patient is in unsatisfactory control (i.e., an FPG concentration ≥130 mg/dl 2–3 weeks after the final dose increase or an A1C level ≥7.0% 3 months after the last evaluation), combination oral therapy with an SU should be started.

Incremental step doses and maximal final doses. Metformin is marketed in tablets containing 500, 850, and 1,000 mg of the drug or in an extended-release form containing 500, 750, and 1,000 mg. The extended-release forms may have fewer GI adverse events. The original studies with the 500-mg tablets suggested that the maximal dose was 2,500 mg. A subsequent dose-response study revealed that there was no additional effect over 2,000 mg. Therefore, if the 500-mg tablet is used, there are usually only three steps (the usual starting dose is 500 mg twice a day), and the patient should take the tablets only twice daily. If the 850-mg tablet is used, there are also only three steps, and the patient takes the tablets three times a day with each meal. If the 1,000-mg tablets are used, there are two steps: 1,000 mg once daily and 1,000 mg twice daily. The extended-release forms need to be taken only once daily and are recommended by the manufacturers to be ingested with the evening meal or at bedtime. The starting dose is either 750 or 1,000 mg, with only a one-step increase for the 1,000-mg tablet (or two 500-mg tablets) to a maximal dose of 2,000 mg or a two-step increase for the 750-mg tablet to a maximal dose of 2,250 mg. Table 5 describes the dosing schedule of various metformin tablet sizes.

Contraindications.

- Renal insufficiency–serum creatinine >1.4 mg/dl for women and >1.5 mg/dl for men if estimated glomerular filtration rate (eGFR) not available; if available, eGFR <30 ml/min/1.73 m^2 (stage 4 kidney disease); use with caution if eGFR 30–50 ml/min/1.73 m^2 (stage 3 kidney disease) (16).
- Hepatic dysfunction: alanine transaminase (ALT) or aspartate transaminase (AST) >3 times normal
- History of alcoholism or binge drinking
- Acute or chronic metabolic acidosis
- Patients >80 years of age (if eGFR is not available)

Discontinuation. The drug should be temporarily discontinued until the following circumstances are no longer present: *1*) acute myocardial infarction, *2*) intravenous contrast material (dye study) and serum creatinine returns to normal or eGFR returns to ≥30 ml/min/1.73 m^2, *3*) major surgery, or *4*) severe infection.

Serious adverse events. Lactic acidosis can occur rarely in patients taking metformin. If this should happen, the mortality is ~20%. Just about all cases have occurred in patients in whom the drug was contraindicated, the great majority of whom had marked renal insufficiency.

Table 5. Metformin Dosing Schedule

Total Dose (mg)	Before Breakfast	Before Lunch	Before Supper
500	500	—	—
1,000[a]	500	—	500
1,500	500	—	1,000[b]
2,000	1,000	—	1,000
OR			
850	850	—	—
1,700	850	—	850
2,550	850	850	850
OR			
Extended Release			
500			500[c]
750[a]	—	—	750[c]
1,000[a]			1,000[c]
1,500			1,500[c]
2,000			2,000[c]
2,250			2,250[c]

Immediate-release forms are in 500-, 850-, and 1,000-mg tablets; extended-release forms are in 500-, 750-, and 1,000-mg tablets. [a]Usual starting dose. [b]Given with largest meal to minimize GI adverse events. [c]Given at bedtime.

SULFONYLUREA AGENTS AND GLINIDES

Mechanism of action. SUs and glinides increase insulin secretion by sensitizing the pancreatic β-cell to respond more vigorously to glucose and amino acids, the usual stimuli.

Principles of use. Starting doses are listed in Table 6. Although second-generation agents (glyburide, glipizide, glimepiride) are commonly used today, two first-generation agents (chlorpropamide, tolazamide) are equally effective, whereas two others (tolbutamide, acetohexImide) are less so. The FPG concentration should be measured ~2–3 weeks after starting an SU and after each dose change. As with metformin, the short-term goal is to achieve a value of <130 mg/dl. If that goal is not achieved, the dose of the SU is increased in one-step increments (see Incremental Step Doses below) until either the goal is met or the maximal dose of the SU is reached. When an FPG concentration of <130 mg/dl is achieved, an A1C level and an FPG concentration should be measured 3 months later.

The long-term goal is to achieve an A1C level of <7.0% in the absence of unexplained hypoglycemia. (Unexplained hypoglycemia is described under Insulin below.) When this goal is achieved, A1C levels and FPG concentrations can be measured every 3 months. If measurements of fasting glucose concentrations by the patient are considered reliable, the average of 3 days of consecutive values may be substituted for a laboratory-measured value. All glucose meters introduced in recent years are calibrated to give plasma levels. Fingerstick blood samples reflect capillary glucose concentrations that are similar to the values measured in the laboratory from a venipuncture sample as long as the patient is in the fasting state. (Random and postprandial values are higher in capillary samples, the difference depending on how long ago the patient ate and the carbohydrate content of the meal.) Whenever FPG concentrations are mentioned in these protocols, measurements of fasting glucose concentrations on 3 consecutive days by reliable patients can be substituted for the laboratory-measured value.

If the maximal dose of the SU is reached (plus metformin unless contraindicated), and the FPG concentration 2–3 weeks later is ≥180 mg/dl or an A1C level 3 months later is ≥7.0%, pioglitazone should be added if not contraindicated. If pioglitazone is contraindicated, consider adding either an oral DPP-4 inhibitor or an injectable incretin analog.

If the FPG concentration 2–3 weeks after the maximal dose of the SU is reached is 130–179 mg/dl, the A1C level measured 3 months later drives the decision whether or not to add a third medication. Some patients taking an SU will have a moderately elevated FPG concentration but an A1C level <7.0%, presumably because the SU via enhanced insulin secretion keeps the glucose levels reasonably low during the day even though they start out >130 mg/dl. Stress diet and exercise during this period, so that the patient can avoid adding the third medication.

Starting and maximal doses. ***All patients starting an SU or a glinide must be taught the signs, symptoms, and treatment of hypoglycemia.*** The starting and maximal doses of the SUs and glinides are shown in Table 6.

Glinides. Repaglinide and nateglinide are drugs that also stimulate β-cells to secrete more insulin. They bind to a different part of the same receptor to which the SUs bind. The difference is that the β-cells respond more quickly to

Table 6. Starting and Maximal Doses of the SUs and Glinides

Generic Name	Brand Name	Starting Dose[a]	Maximal Dose
Tolbutamide	Orinase	1,000[b]	3,000
Acetohexamide	Dymelor	250	1,500
Tolazamide	Tolinase	100	1,000
Chlorpropamide[c]	Diabinese	100	750
Glyburide[c]	Micronase, DiaBeta	5	20
Glyburide (micronized)[c]	Glynase	3	12
Glipizide	Glucotrol	10	40
Glipizide (extended release)	Glucotrol XL	5	20
Glimepiride	Amaryl	2	8
Repaglinide	Prandin	1[d]	Usually 12[d]
Nateglinide	Starlix	120[e]	360

[a]Smaller starting doses are often recommended, but in my experience, higher doses are almost always needed. [b]Initial doses given before breakfast and supper with subsequent step introduced before lunch. [c]Should not be a first-line agent in patients >65 years of age; the Expert Committee doesn't recommend them at all because of increased risk of hypoglycemia compared with other SUs. [d]Maximum dose of 16 mg is 4 mg per meal (if a fourth meal is eaten). If a meal is missed, that dose (whatever the amount) should be omitted. A dose is usually not taken for a small bedtime snack. [e]Before each meal.

glinides and only for a short period of time leading to rapid increases in insulin levels that quickly return to baseline levels. Therefore, there is somewhat less hypoglycemia in patients taking glinides compared with SUs. These drugs are advantageous for patients who have irregular eating patterns. A disadvantage is that they must be taken before each meal, usually three times a day.

Incremental step doses. The dosing schedules for the SUs and glinides are shown in Table 7. (Manufacturers' recommended initial doses smaller than those in Table 6 are in parentheses.)

Table 7. Dosing Schedule for SUs and Glinides

Total Dose (mg)	Before Breakfast	Before Lunch	Before Supper
Second-Generation Drugs			
Glyburide (Micronase, DiaBeta)			
(1.25)	(1.25)		
(2.5)	(2.5)	—	—
5	5	—	—
10	10	—	—
15	10	—	5
20	10	—	10
Micronized Glyburide (Glynase)			
(1.5)	(1.5)	—	—
3	3	—	—
6	6	—	—
9	6	—	3
12	6	—	6
Glipizide (Glucotrol)			
(2.5)	(2.5)		
(5)	(5)	—	—
10	10	—	—
20	20	—	—
30	20	—	10
40	20	—	20
Extended-release glipizide (Glucotrol XL)			
(2.5)	(2.5)	—	—
5	5	—	—
10	10	—	—
20	20	—	—
Glimepiridea (Amaryl)			
(1)	(1)	—	—
2	2	—	—
4	4	—	—
6	6	—	—
8	8	—	—
First-Generation Drugs			
Tolbutamide (Orinase)			
(500)	(250)	—	(250)
1,000	500	—	500
1,500	500	500	500
2,000	1,000	—	1,000
3,000	1,000	1,000	1,000

Total Dose (mg)	Before Breakfast	Before Lunch	Before Supper
Acetohexamide (Dymelor)			
250	250	—	—
500	500	—	—
750	750	—	—
1,000	1,000	—	—
1,500	1,000	—	500
Tolazamide (Tolinase)			
100	100	—	—
250	250	—	—
500	500	—	—
750	500	—	250
1,000	500	—	500
Chlorpropamide[a] (Diabinese)			
100	100	—	—
250	250	—	—
500	500	—	—
750	750	—	—
Glinides			
Repaglinide[b] (Prandin)			
(1.5)	(0.5)	(0.5)	(0.5)
3	1.0	1.0	1.0
6	2.0	2.0	2.0
12	4.0	4.0	4.0
Nateglinide (Starlix)			
360	120	120	120

[a]Can be taken at any time of day. [b]Maximum dose of 16 mg is 4 mg per meal (if a fourth meal is eaten).

Combination pills. There are several medications that are combined in one pill in various doses (all given in milligrams):

Glucovance (glyburide/metformin) (available as generic): 1.25/250; 2.5/500; 5.0/500
Metaglip (glipizide/metformin) (available as generic): 2.5/250; 2.5/500; 5.0/500
Avandamet (rosiglitazone/metformin): 2/500; 4/500
Avandaryl (rosiglitazone/glimepiride): 4/1; 4/2; 4/4; 8/2; 8/4
Actoplus Met (pioglitazone/metformin): 15/500; 15/850
Duetact (pioglitazone/glimepiride): 30/2; 30/4
Janumet (sitagliptin/metformin): 50/500; 50/1000

There are no added clinical advantages to these combinations. They are more expensive than the individual generics, and titrating the doses up can be more difficult. Using them contradicts the cost-effective principle of starting with a generic medication, increasing it until an appropriate response is seen, or, if a maximal (tolerated) dose is reached, adding a second medication and following the same procedure. An exception to this statement may occur in patients who have a copayment for each medication prescribed. In that case, a combination pill may save them money.

THIAZOLIDINEDIONES (GLITAZONES)

Mechanism of action. TZDs bind to a nuclear receptor (called the peroxisome proliferator–activated receptor γ, or PPAR-γ). This binding results in activation of a gene or genes that increase(s) glucose utilization (probably by increasing glucose transport) in muscle and fat tissue. In this manner, TZDs decrease peripheral insulin resistance, which is an important characteristic of type 2 diabetes. They also have a more minor effect on reducing hepatic insulin resistance leading to decreased hepatic glucose production.

Clinical use. The U.S. Food and Drug Administration (FDA) has approved two TZDs (rosiglitazone [Avandia] and pioglitazone [Actos]) for use in type 2 diabetic patients. (They are not indicated for type 1 diabetic patients.) They can be used as monotherapy, in combination with other oral antihyperglycemic drugs or with insulin. TZDs take 2–4 weeks before an effect can be seen (consistent with their mechanism of action affecting gene expression) with a maximal effect not evident for 3–4 months. Rosiglitazone is marketed in 2-, 4-, and 8-mg tablets. Pioglitazone is marketed in 15-, 30-, and 45-mg tablets. Because a maximum response to a glitazone may take up to 4 months, if a patient starts with a submaximal dose, planning to increase it if an inadequate response is documented, it may take the better part of a year before knowing whether the patient will have an adequate response to the glitazone. For this reason, start the patient with the maximum dose—8 mg once a day for rosiglitazone and 45 mg once a day for pioglitazone. With this approach, you will know in 4 months whether the patient will have an adequate response (see below) to the glitazone. Because all of these patients will be on a maximal dose of an SU, measure the FPG concentration 2 months after starting the glitazone to ascertain that the patient is not hypoglycemic. If the FPG concentration is <70 mg/dl (or if the patient is having hypoglycemic episodes), the dose of the SU, not the glitazone, should be reduced.

If the next step is either exenatide (see Incretins below) or insulin, which is often the case because glitazones are frequently the last of triple oral therapy added, accept a 4-month target A1C level of <7.5%. This level is acceptable at this juncture because both exenatide and insulin need to be injected. There is also a high chance of exenatide causing nausea, at least initially. Furthermore, insulin therapy requires major lifestyle changes, including SMBG, less flexibility in eating and exercise patterns, and the potential for hypoglycemia. Five studies in over 2,000 type 1 (17–19) and type 2 (20,21) diabetic patients followed for 4–9 years showed that there was only a slight increase in the development or progression of microvascular complications of diabetes if the average A1C level was maintained between 7.0 and 8.0% (and no increase in these complications if the average values were between 6.0 and 7.0%). If the A1C level rises above 7.5% on subsequent testing, I discontinue the glitazone and add either exenatide or bedtime NPH or glargine insulin.

Both rosiglitazone and pioglitazone have been shown to lower A1C levels when added to patients poorly controlled on high doses of insulin. Consider adding one of the glitazones when patients on a total dose of insulin exceeding 80 units/day remain poorly controlled. However, keep in mind the increased risk of edema, heart failure, and more weight gain with the combination of a glitazone and insulin. It is important that patients be willing and able to furnish SMBG values when a glitazone is added, because lower glucose levels necessitating a decrease of insulin doses may occur. Try to anticipate these changes before frank hypoglycemia occurs.

Adverse effects. Troglitazone (Rezulin), the first approved TZD, was removed from the market because of rare, but sometimes fatal, hepatic failure. These episodes were preceded by elevations in hepatic transaminases, especially ALT. Although there were no differences in increases in ALT levels between patients receiving placebo and those receiving either rosiglitazone or pioglitazone during preapproval clinical studies, because of the structural similarity among the three TZDs, the FDA initially recommended that patients receiving the two new ones also have their hepatic function monitored until more experience with them was obtained. Based on the post-marketing extensive experience with both rosiglitazone and pioglitazone and the lack of evidence of hepatic dysfunction attributed to these drugs, the FDA removed the requirement for ongoing liver function testing in the absence of another clinical reason for it. However, the FDA recommends that ALT levels be measured before starting rosiglitazone or pioglitazone. Neither drug should be started if ALT levels are >2.5 times the upper limit of normal, and both should be discontinued if values exceed 3 times the upper limit of normal.

TZDs increase the plasma volume slightly by increasing fluid retention. This increased plasma volume results in a clinically insignificant lowering of the hematocrit and hemoglobin level and the white blood cell count and may help account for some of the weight gain noted in some patients. The increase in fluid retention may also cause or worsen edema, as well as heart failure, in individuals who already have either condition or are prone to getting either one. These drugs were not studied in patients with New York Heart Association Class III or IV cardiac status and should be avoided in these individuals. Therefore, TZDs should be used with caution in patients with a history of edema. TZD use is not advised in patients who have edema already present or a history of heart failure.

If peripheral edema occurs, the dose of the glitazone can be reduced (halved to 4 mg once a day for rosiglitazone and decreased to 30 mg once a day for pioglitazone) or discontinued (and another treatment added). If the dose of the glitazone is reduced and edema persists, discontinue the drug. When glitazones are discontinued, there are three choices: substituting exenatide, bedtime insulin, or possibly a DPP-4 inhibitor (see Incretins). The latter might be tried because there is no dose titration, a maximal effect on the FPG concentration is seen within 1 month, and the side effect profile is so benign (2). Keep in mind that just as the onset of action of glitazones is delayed, so is the waning of their effect. Therefore, although initially it may seem that the DPP-4 inhibitor is maintaining the patient in satisfactory control, this may not be the case several months later.

Whenever the A1C level exceeds 7.5%, exenatide or bedtime insulin should be instituted. A head-to-head comparison (22) between glargine insulin and exenatide added to oral anti-hyperglycemic drugs revealed equal effectiveness in lowering A1C levels. As might be expected, fasting glucose concentrations decreased more with insulin, while postprandial concentrations decreased more with the GLP-1 agonist. Patients receiving insulin gained weight, while those individuals injecting exenatide lost weight. The weight loss, non-necessity of SMBG, and the much lower risk of hypoglycemia associated with the GLP-1 agonist might be added advantages.

Several recent studies have shown that glitazones are associated with decreased bone mineral density (23,24) and increased fractures in both men and women, although there is more of a risk in women (25,26).

Lipid effects. TZDs have varying effects on lipids. Total cholesterol and LDL cholesterol concentrations are increased by both rosiglitazone and pioglitazone, but more so with rosiglitazone. High density lipoprotein (HDL) cholesterol concentrations are also increased by both glitazones, but more so with pioglitazone. Neither the total cholesterol/HDL cholesterol nor the LDL cholesterol/HDL cholesterol ratios changed appreciably in patients receiving rosiglitazone and pioglitazone. Moreover, the LDL particle shifted from a more atherogenic small dense particle size to a less atherogenic large fluffy one with both glitazones. Finally, fasting triglyceride concentrations were decreased by pioglitazone, but not by rosiglitazone.

Drug interactions. The following drug interactions between the TZDs and other drugs have been studied. There are no drug interactions between rosiglitazone and oral contraceptive agents, glyburide, digoxin, warfarin, nifidipine, metformin, acarbose, ranitidine, or ethanol. There are no drug interactions between pioglitazone and digoxin, warfarin, metformin, or glipizide. The effect on oral contraceptive agents has not been studied. In vitro studies showed that ketoconazole significantly inhibited the metabolism of pioglitazone. Therefore, pending the availability of additional data, patients receiving ketoconazole concomitantly with pioglitazone should be evaluated more frequently with respect to glycemic control.

Miscellaneous. Dose adjustments of the two glitazones are not necessary in the elderly or in patients with renal insufficiency. Some anovulatory women with the polycystic ovary syndrome (PCOS) have ovulated, and a few have conceived when receiving metformin. This is presumably due to the reduction of insulin resistance, which characterizes PCOS, leading to a reduction of hyperandrogenism and improvement in gonadotropin secretion. Recent small studies have shown the same effect of the glitazones in women with PCOS. Because glitazones cause intrauterine growth retardation in animal studies, they should be discontinued immediately if conception occurs in women with PCOS. Appropriate contraception is advised for those women receiving glitazones (or metformin) who do not wish to become pregnant.

Which glitazone? Although disputed by some (27), several recent meta-analyses have suggested that rosiglitazone is associated with a slight increase in cardiac events (28,29). This led to the decision made at the consensus conference not to recommend the use of rosiglitazone (1). However, an in-depth analysis by the FDA, presented at the annual meeting of the American Diabetes Association in June 2008, and a multicenter, open-label trial in nearly 4,500 patients (30) did not substantiate the claim that rosiglitazone had a detrimental effect on CVD events. On the other hand, pioglitazone may actually have a beneficial effect on CVD events (31,32). Pioglitazone is also preferred because of its more favorable effect on lipids.

INCRETINS

Background. It was shown nearly 50 years ago that glucose given by mouth elicits a greater insulin response than amounts given intravenously that yield similar plasma glucose concentrations reached after oral glucose. The difference in insulin levels between oral and intravenous administration (despite similar plasma glucose concentrations) is called the “incretin effect” and was postulated to involve factors secreted by the gastrointestinal tract after oral glucose ingestion. One of these factors is the hormone GLP-1. Within minutes after starting a meal, the L-cells in the distal ileum secrete GLP-1. Although food has obviously not reached the distal ileum at this time, K-cells in the upper duodenum signal the brain (via vagus pathways) to stimulate the L-cells to secrete GLP-1. The half-life of GLP-1 in the circulation is only 2 min because the enzyme DPP-4 quickly inactivates the hormone. Although GLP-1 and glucagon share some homology (hence the similarity of their names), their actions are much different. Glucagon is a counterregulatory hormone that increases hepatic glucose production. In contrast, GLP-1 inhibits glucagon secretion, stimulates insulin secretion in a glucose-dependent manner, slows gastric emptying, and suppresses appetite. The glucose-dependent aspect of stimulating insulin secretion means that the increase in insulin release only occurs when glucose concentrations are elevated, not when they are normal.

Incretin analogs. The saliva of the Gila monster (a large lizard) contains a compound, marketed as exenatide (Byetta), that shares homology with GLP-1. One of the differences between the two molecules occurs at the site where DPP-4 inactivates GLP-1. Therefore, DPP-4 does not inactivate exenatide, which has a half-life of many hours after subcutaneous injection. By virtue of the ability of exenatide to suppress glucagon (which is normally suppressed after eating, but not in people with diabetes), to stimulate insulin secretion, and to delay gastric emptying, the postprandial rise of glucose is blunted. Fasting glucose concentrations also decrease but not as much as postprandial concentrations. Exenatide also decreases appetite, resulting in weight loss in many patients, which in turn increases insulin sensitivity, also resulting in improved diabetes control. Based on the criteria for selecting drugs discussed earlier, it is recommended to use exenatide after triple oral therapy has failed (Figure 3). If the A1C level exceeds 7.5% at any time after 4 months of treatment, exenatide should be discontinued, and insulin should be introduced.

Up to 30% of patients receiving exenatide experience nausea that is usually mild and often gradually disappears over several weeks to a month. The weight loss is slightly greater in these patients but is also seen in patients without nausea. On average, weight loss (~10 lb) has been maintained for over 1 year. Because of the glucose dependence of insulin secretion, exenatide by itself does not cause hypoglycemia. However, because patients who are also receiving an SU may experience hypoglycemia, the dose of this oral drug should be halved when exenatide is started. If hypoglycemia does not occur, the dose should be maximized again. Exenatide has been associated with rare cases of pancreatitis.

Exenatide is injected just before breakfast and supper. It is supplied in prefilled pens, either 5 or 10 μg per dose. Each pen contains 60 doses (30-day supply). The initial dose is 5 μg twice daily for the first month, increasing to

10 µg twice daily, the maximal approved dose. If breakfast or supper is missed, exenatide should not be given. The 5 µg dose can be used if the glycemic response is optimal or the patient cannot tolerate the nausea at the 10-µg dose.

DPP-4 inhibitors. Compounds that inhibit the DPP-4 enzyme should allow endogenous GLP-1 to remain active for longer periods of time. A single oral dose of sitagliptin (Januvia), the first marketed DPP-4 inhibitor, maintains its inhibition of the enzyme for >24 h and thereby increases the postprandial response of GLP-1 for >24 h. As with exenatide, FPG concentrations are decreased somewhat but not nearly as much as postprandial concentrations. The maximal lowering of FPG concentrations occurs by 3 weeks with no further decline. Sitagliptin has a benign side effect profile with no increase in GI symptoms compared with control subjects in clinical trials. Unlike exenatide, it is weight neutral. There was a slight increase in nasopharyngitis in patients taking sitagliptin in one clinical trial compared with control subjects, but no difference was seen when all patients taking sitagliptin in clinical trials were compared with subjects taking placebos. In postmarketing experience with sitagliptin, rare cases of hypersensitivity (anaphylaxis, urticaria, cutaneous vasculitis), exfoliative skin conditions including Stevens-Johnson syndrome, and pancreatitis were reported. Because these reactions are reported voluntarily from a population of uncertain size, it is generally not possible to reliably estimate their frequency or establish a causal relationship to drug exposure. Because GLP-1 stimulates insulin secretion in a glucose-dependent manner, sitagliptin also does not cause hypoglycemia. The dose of sitagliptin is 100 mg once a day. Because ~80% is excreted unchanged in the urine, the dose must be reduced in patients with renal insufficiency. In moderate renal insufficiency, the dose is 50 mg/day in men with serum creatinine levels of 1.8–3.0 mg/dl and in women with creatinine levels of 1.6–2.5 mg/dl. In severe renal insufficiency, men with serum creatinine levels >3.0 mg/dl and women with levels of >2.5 mg/dl should receive 25 mg/day. If glomerular filtration rates are estimated (most likely) or measured, moderate renal insufficiency is defined as a creatinine clearance of ≥30–50 ml/min/1.73 m2, and severe renal insufficiency as <30 ml/min/1.73 m2.

A new DPP-4 inhibitor, saxagliptin (Onglyza), was just approved by the Federal Drug Administration. It seems very similar to sitagliptin in its efficacy. During the clinical trials, its adverse event profile was benign. It is taken once a day, 5.0 mg in patients with eGFR values >50 ml/min, and 2.5 mg in individuals with moderate (30–50 ml/min) or severe (<30 ml/min) renal insufficiency.

α-GLUCOSIDASE INHIBITORS

Mechanism of action. α-Glucosidases are the enzymes that break down carbohydrates to glucose, which is then absorbed from the small intestine into the circulation. Therefore, inhibition of these enzymes delays the absorption of glucose until further down in the small intestine, which in turn flattens out the postprandial rise of blood glucose concentrations.

Principles of use. Two α-glucosidase inhibitors are approved by the FDA—acarbose (Precose) and miglitol (Glyset). The recommended initial dose for both is 25 mg given orally at the start (with the first bite) of each main meal, and the dosage is gradually increased. However, some patients may benefit by starting at 25 mg once daily to minimize GI adverse events (see Adverse Events below) and gradually increasing the frequency of administration to three times a day before each meal. In that case, either drug should be started at 25 mg with a meal for 1–2 weeks, increased to 25 mg with a second meal for another 1–2 weeks, and finally increased to 25 mg with the third meal if the GI side effects can be tolerated by the patient. If the level of control is unsatisfactory, the dose is gradually increased to 50 mg before each meal (GI side effects permitting). Although the largest impact of the α-glucosidase inhibitors is seen on the 1- to 2-h postprandial glucose concentration, this test may be difficult to schedule accurately and is greatly influenced by the carbohydrate content of the meal. Therefore, one value may not accurately represent the patient's glycemic status. An A1C level 3 months after reaching a stable dose can be used to decide whether to continue to increase the dose. (100 mg three times a day is the maximal dose in patients weighing >60 kg and 50 mg three times a day in patients weighing <60 kg.) Alternatively, the dose can be increased gradually to the maximum (or maximally tolerated) to derive its greatest benefit. Increasing progressively to the maximum (or maximally tolerated) dose is preferable, in my view, because if one has to wait 3 months after a submaximal dose is stabilized to evaluate the glycemic status with an A1C level, it may take up to a year with gradually increasing doses to determine whether an α-glucosidase inhibitor will be effective enough.

Adverse effects. The major side effect is flatulence, although a few patients may also have diarrhea. These side effects will decrease over time, especially if small doses are used initially and increased slowly, as described above. Approximately 20% of patients will have persistent flatulence and may not be able to tolerate the drug. Elevation of hepatic transaminases (ALT, AST) may rarely occur. These abnormalities almost always reverse when the drug is discontinued. The drug is not recommended to be used in patients with creatinine concentrations of >2 mg/dl (because no long-term trials in diabetic patients with this level of renal insufficiency have been conducted) or with intestinal disorders.

Hypoglycemia. The α-glucosidase inhibitors *will not* cause hypoglycemia when used as monotherapy. Hypoglycemia may occur, however, when the drug is added to an SU or insulin. In this case, the hypoglycemia is due, of course, to one of the latter drugs. If this should occur, *hypoglycemia must be treated with either dextrose (glucose) tablets or milk*. The α-glucosidase inhibitors do not inhibit the enzyme that breaks down the carbohydrate in milk (i.e., lactose to glucose and galactose, which is why lactose intolerance is not an adverse effect of the drugs). However, these drugs will delay the absorption of other disaccharides and more complex carbohydrates, which is why these sources of carbohydrate should not be used to treat hypoglycemia. Because glucose is a monosaccharide, its absorption is not affected by α-glucosidase inhibitors.

TREATMENT OF MARKEDLY SYMPTOMATIC, NEWLY DIAGNOSED TYPE 2 DIABETIC PATIENTS

First, markedly symptomatic patients are defined here as individuals with increased urination and thirst occurring every several hours, day and night, and often associated with weight loss in the presence of increased appetite, blurring of vision, and sometimes fungal infections. Patients recently diagnosed with type 2 diabetes can be successfully treated with maximal (<65 years of age) or half-maximal (≥65 years of age) doses of an SU. In my hands, this therapy (33) has been effective in >90% of over 200 such type 2 diabetic patients, even though their glucose levels can exceed 500 mg/dl and they can be ketotic, some with bicarbonate levels as low as 15 mEq/l. Of course, insulin therapy is also appropriate in these patients, but using maximal doses of an SU is much easier for patients and physicians alike and just as effective in almost all cases. If these are truly recently diagnosed type 2 diabetic patients, they will start to respond, at least to some extent, to a maximal dose of an SU within a week or two. These markedly symptomatic patients have had weeks to months of marked hyperglycemia so that another several weeks before they are brought under control is not too detrimental. It must be emphasized that this approach applies only to newly (or recently, within the past 6 months or so) diagnosed patients. Patients with a longer duration of diagnosed type 2 diabetes will often not have enough β-cell function left to respond sufficiently to an insulin secretagogue.

Second, clinical clues suggesting that the patient has type 2 diabetes are *1*) obese (BMI ≥30 kg/m^2) or at least overweight (BMI 26.0–29.9 kg/m^2), *2*) ethnic minority, and *3*) positive family history in one or more first-degree relatives. If patients have all of these, it is very likely that they have type 2 diabetes.

Third, because all patients with type 2 diabetes should be taking metformin, this medication could also be started and the dose adjusted upward as described above.

Fourth, principles of SU therapy are as follows: Most physicians start insulin, usually in the hospital, but sometimes as outpatients. This is not necessary. In those few patients who do not respond adequately to high doses of an SU and progressively increasing doses of metformin, insulin may be necessary. If so, it can be started several weeks to several months later in an outpatient setting under less "emergent" conditions. A flow chart guiding the treatment of markedly symptomatic type 2 diabetic patients is provided at the end of the Glycemia Algorithm. In recently diagnosed patients, the initial dose of the SU often needs to be tapered, because lowering glucose concentrations increases insulin secretion (i.e., reversal of glucose toxicity on the β-cell).

PRAMLINTIDE (SYMLIN)

Background. Amylin is co-secreted with insulin from the pancreatic β-cell. Amylin self-aggregates (sticks together to form clumps) and adheres to surfaces. By changing several amino acids in its structure, the resulting molecule (pramlintide) does not self-aggregate and is much easier to work with. Although the physiological function of amylin is unknown, pramlintide has many of the properties of GLP-1. It suppresses glucagon secretion, slows gastric emptying, and decreases appetite (but does not stimulate insulin secretion).

Clinical use. Pramlintide is injected (in a separate syringe at sites at least 2 inches away from the insulin injection site) at mealtimes in type 1 diabetic patients and insulin-requiring type 2 diabetic patients. Although there is a small significant effect on lowering FPG concentrations, its major effect is on postprandial glucose levels, as would be expected from its effects described in Background above. Many patients also lose weight. The initial dose in type 1 diabetic patients is 15 μg before each major meal. Because of the possibility of nausea (see Adverse Reactions), the insulin dose should be reduced by 50% and adjusted upward as indicated by glucose monitoring. If there is no significant nausea with 15 μg before each meal, the pramlintide dose is increased by 15-μg increments before each meal every 3–7 days until preprandial doses of 60 μg are reached. In insulin-requiring type 2 diabetic patients, the insulin dose is also decreased by 50% (and adjusted upward as dictated by glucose monitoring), but the initial dose of pramlintide is 60 μg before each major meal and increased in one step to maximal doses of 120 μg, nausea permitting.

Adverse effects. Approximately one-third of patients will experience significant nausea, which usually improves over time. It often recurs after each dose increase, but in the clinical trials, <10% withdrew because of nausea. (Remember, however, that these subjects are especially motivated, and nausea may be more of a problem in the real-world setting.) In the clinical trials in which insulin doses were not changed initially, hypoglycemia was an issue, which is why an initial dose decrease of insulin (with subsequent upward titration as indicated) is recommended.

SELF-MONITORING OF BLOOD GLUCOSE

SMBG is extremely important for adjusting insulin doses, and its use will be described in some detail in the insulin sections below. However, there is very little evidence demonstrating that SMBG in non–insulin-treated patients improves glycemia. A few observational studies show that SMBG in these patients is associated with slightly lower A1C levels than in individuals who did not perform SMBG. However, this association is likely due to patient self-selection, e.g., those with healthier lifestyles are more likely to test (34), or to physician self-selection, e.g., they are more likely to order SMBG in newly diagnosed type 2 diabetic patients in whom initial treatment always improves glycemia. Figure 4 shows a negative correlation between A1C levels and the number of SMBG tests performed per day in insulin-requiring type 2 patients, as might be expected, but shows a positive correlation in patients not taking insulin. The latter is related to another aspect of physician self-selection, in that patients uncontrolled in the

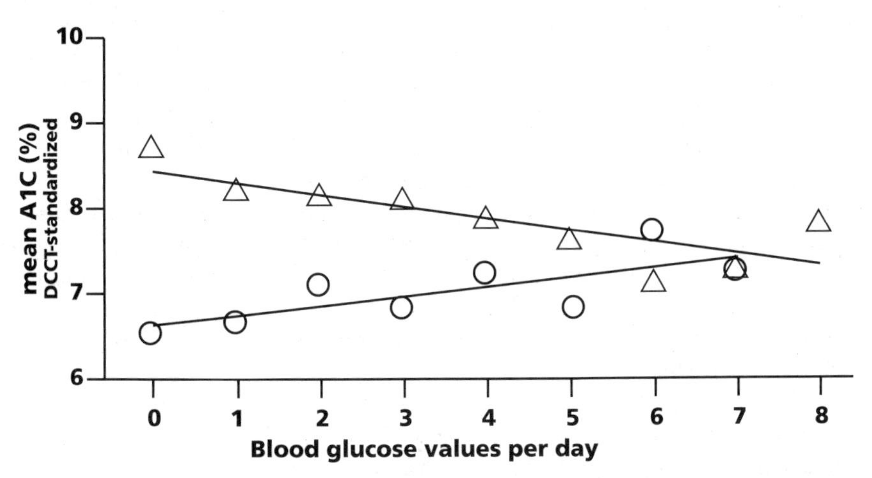

Figure 4. Effect of SMBG in patients with type 2 diabetes treated with insulin (△, *n* = 2,021) or with oral antidiabetes drugs and/or diet (○, *n* = 2,988). Data are adjusted for age, diabetes duration, gender, BMI–*z*-score, treatment center, and year of therapy. Reprinted with permission from Schutt et al. (43).

years after diagnosis are more likely to be asked to carry out more testing to bring them under control. Causation needs to be evaluated in randomized clinical trials; observational studies can only be hypothesis generating.

Randomized clinical trials do not support the use of SMBG in non–insulin-treated diabetic patients for improving glycemia. A review of 12 randomized clinical trials revealed that in all five of the trials showing a significant lowering of A1C levels in patients performing SMBG compared with control subjects, the SMBG group received more intensive education and/or treatment than the control group (35). Since that review, five more large randomized clinical trials did not demonstrate lowering of A1C levels in patients performing SMBG compared with their control subjects, and a few revealed more anxiety and depression in subjects who tested.

With a little reflection, it is not surprising that SMBG has not improved glycemic outcomes in non–insulin-treated patients. For SMBG to be helpful, patients must act on the results. Patients taking insulin can adjust their preprandial doses. For non–insulin-treated patients, only adjusting doses of a glinide or an α-glucosidase inhibitor (each of which has only ~1% market share of oral antidiabetes drugs in the U.S.) will have an effect. Patients could change the carbohydrate content or delay the meal or engage in increased exercise after the meal. However, these behavioral changes are either not being done or are ineffective (probably the former), as evidenced by the negative results of the randomized clinical trials in non–insulin-treated patients.

SMBG has the potential to educate and motivate non–insulin-treated patients. SMBG values could educate patients on the effects of carbohydrate content and size of meals, and high values could motivate them to follow prescribed diets and to change a sedentary lifestyle to a more active one. To maximize the education, patients should perform SMBG before and between 1 and 2 h after the same meal to isolate the glycemic response to that meal. For motivational purposes, postprandial values (preferably after the largest meal) should be measured. Regrettably, the overwhelming majority of tests in these patients are preprandial ones, which would have much less effect on educating and motivating patients. A more fundamental barrier for SMBG to improve glycemia in non–insulin-treated patients is the general difficulty of people changing their behaviors.

SMBG is very expensive (35). In the absence of much evidence attesting to its benefit in patients not taking insulin, it is not part of the Glycemia Algorithms for these patients. In a study in which a nurse treated over 350 patients in a county clinic by following these algorithms and achieved a mean A1C level of 7.0% (36), the mean A1C level in subjects not taking insulin who also did not perform SMBG was 6.7%. Therefore, SMBG is not necessary to reach the ADA goal in non–insulin-treated patients as long as timely appropriate treatment decisions are being made (37).

INSULIN

The general approach in using insulin is to craft an insulin regimen around the patient's usual eating and exercise patterns rather than to impose an insulin regimen that requires patients to change their lifestyle to accommodate it. This approach can sometimes be quite challenging, e.g., in patients who work evening or overnight shifts during the week but not on weekends. But in the final analysis, this approach is the only way for these patients to control glycemia without having diabetes markedly disrupt their lives. The following five questions should be asked of every insulin-treated patient when adjusting their doses:

1. What are the doses of insulin currently being taken? The reason for this question is obvious.
2. What is the pattern and frequency of SMBG? When is SMBG being carried out, and how often at each time? Preprandial and before-bedtime snack are the usual times recommended. (Every patient taking insulin should take a small bedtime snack to minimize overnight hypoglycemia.) If preprandial values are on-target, and the A1C level is still >7.0%, 1- to 2-h postprandial glucose concentrations should be measured. In that case, these postprandial tests substitute for the subsequent preprandial tests, e.g., postprandial breakfast tests replace the preprandial lunch tests, which would be in the target range before asking for postprandial testing.
3. What are the values at each time of testing? As discussed below, the results at each time reflect a different component of the insulin prescription. Therefore, daily, weekly, or monthly average values are not helpful in adjusting insulin doses.
4. What are the frequency and pattern of hypoglycemia? If hypoglycemia occurs less than once or twice a month, it probably does not need to be specifically addressed. If it occurs more frequently, its pattern (i.e., when it occurs) may give a clue as to how to address it. For example, if hypoglycemia usually occurs between breakfast and lunch, the dose of short- or rapid-acting insulin taken before breakfast probably needs to be decreased. Hypoglycemia occurring overnight may necessitate starting a bedtime snack (if that is not already part of the patient's usual eating pattern); reducing the evening NPH, glargine, or detemir insulin dose; or possibly moving the NPH injection from before supper to bedtime.
5. Is hypoglycemia explained or unexplained? This is extremely important to differentiate. *Explained* hypoglycemia occurs if a meal is delayed or missed or unanticipated exercise takes place. Consistency of lifestyle needs to be stressed in this case. *Unexplained* hypoglycemia occurs in the presence of the patient's usual eating and exercise patterns. In this case, the appropriate insulin dose needs to be adjusted downward.

Many patients will state that they have had episodes of (undocumented) hypoglycemia. It is important for the provider to determine whether these are bona fide hypoglycemic episodes. In addition to deciding whether the symptoms are consistent with hypoglycemia, the key questions to ask are whether the patient ate something at that time, and if so, how long it took to feel better. If the symptoms don't start to improve within 20 min (often much faster) after eating, it is unlikely that this represents true hypoglycemia.

BEDTIME INSULIN AND DAYTIME ORAL ANTIDIABETES DRUGS

Background. In the majority of type 2 diabetic patients, the FPG concentration is the major determinant of the level of glycemia throughout the day. Stated differently, the postprandial rise of glucose concentrations is approximately the same regardless of the preprandial value. Glucose concentrations before lunch and supper are often only slightly higher than before breakfast, i.e., given enough time (4–5 h), the postprandial rise returns to nearly baseline values. Furthermore, the literature shows that multiple-dose insulin regimens did not yield better control than bedtime NPH insulin plus oral antidiabetes drugs when compared for up to 1 year (9–12). Therefore, if the FPG concentration can be lowered appreciably, overall diabetic control is often significantly improved.

Principles of use. The intermediate-acting insulin, NPH, given at bedtime, and two peakless insulins, glargine and detemir, whenever given (see Regimens of Multiple Insulin Injections below), lower the FPG concentration, while the oral antidiabetes drugs control the daytime glucose concentrations. Bedtime insulin is an easy way to introduce insulin therapy to type 2 diabetic patients who have failed oral antidiabetes drugs. There is only one insulin injection, and initially it is necessary to measure only the fasting glucose level. Because the peak effect of the NPH insulin occurs around breakfast time, and glargine and detemir insulins are peakless, there is much less chance of daytime hypoglycemia mediated by exogenous insulin compared with a regimen in which NPH insulin is injected before breakfast or short- or rapid-acting insulin is given before meals. This bedtime-insulin approach gives patients much more flexibility in their eating and exercise patterns during the day. There are somewhat fewer hypoglycemic reactions overnight with glargine and detemir insulin compared with NPH insulin. (However, overnight hypoglycemia is usually not a problem with gradual increases in the doses of NPH insulin, especially if the patient ingests a small bedtime snack.) Although it was postulated that glargine insulin might help in controlling afternoon hyperglycemia compared with bedtime NPH insulin, this has not proved true, regardless of whether glargine insulin was given in the morning or evening (38).

Once the goal FPG target is reached (see below), control throughout the day depends on the oral antidiabetes drugs. Except for adherence to appropriate diet and exercise regimens, the patient can do little to affect daytime control, which at this point is mainly determined by the ability of pancreatic β-cells to secrete insulin. (Some patients may need to know this to avoid self-blame.)

Oral antidiabetes drug. When patients fail combination oral antidiabetes therapy (often an SU, metformin, and a glitazone) and require the addition of insulin to improve glycemic control, bedtime NPH or glargine insulin is started. Discontinuation of glitazone is recommended, and so is maintaining the maximal (tolerated) doses of metformin and the SU. The glitazone should be stopped because with insulin there is not only the likelihood of more weight gain due to fat accumulation, but also the increased possibility of edema due to fluid retention. The increased cost of TZDs might also be a consideration if satisfactory control can be achieved without the glitazone. If bedtime insulin plus maximal (tolerated) doses of metformin and SU does not achieve the target A1C level, addition of a glitazone may be considered before intensifying the insulin regimen.

Goal of therapy. The goal is to lower the FPG concentration measured daily to 70–130 mg/dl.

Initial dose of NPH insulin. The initial dose of bedtime NPH or the peakless insulins depends on whether the patient is overweight/obese or lean, as calculated in Chapter 2. Overweight and obese patients are started on 16 units, and lean patients are started on 10 units. These doses are almost always less than the patient eventually requires but do help avoid potentially discouraging episodes of overnight hypoglycemia initially. If the insulin dose is adjusted appropriately (see Insulin Dose Adjustments below), the appropriate amount is quickly achieved.

Insulin dose adjustments. The dose of bedtime insulin is increased rapidly until the fasting glucose concentration is <150 mg/dl, and then more gradually to reach the appropriate fasting glucose goal. The dose can be increased by 4 units in overweight and obese patients, and 2 units in lean patients whose fasting glucose concentrations remain >200 mg/dl for several days in a row. Increases for fasting glucose concentrations of 150–200 mg/dl for several days in a row can be 2 units and 1 unit, respectively. Some patients can be taught the algorithm in Table 8 to facilitate reaching the initial dose of bedtime insulin.

Table 8. Algorithm for Initial Bedtime Insulin Dose Adjustments

Fasting Glucose for 2 Days in a Row	Increase in Bedtime Insulin Dose (units)	
	Overweight/Obese	Lean
>200 mg/dl	4	2
150–200 mg/dl[a]	2	1

[a]Use this dose increase if the fasting glucose concentration is >200 mg/dl one day and 150–200 mg/dl the next day.

Once the FPG concentration is <150 mg/dl for a week (i.e., at least 4 of 7 days), increase the bedtime insulin dose less frequently to reach the appropriate goal levels. This can be achieved by using 7 days of FPG values to decide on possible dose adjustments. If the majority of values (i.e., at least four of the seven measurements) are >130 mg/dl, increase the dose in overweight/obese and lean patients by 4 and 2 units, respectively, or 10% of the current dose, whichever is greater, until the majority of values are in the target range. If blood glucose values are analyzed over a period longer than 1 week, increase the insulin dose if the majority (i.e., ≥50%) of values are ≥130 mg/dl (e.g., ≥5/10, ≥7/14, ≥11/21, ≥14/28, or ≥50% of the values at any time between 1 and 4 weeks). Glucose values should be analyzed at least every month, and more frequently if possible, when initial doses are being adjusted.

Subsequent follow-up. Once the fasting glucose concentrations are <150 mg/dl, if the patient is taking the maximal dose of an SU, daytime hypoglycemia may occur. Therefore, these patients should measure their glucose concentrations before supper several times a week at this point. Values <80 mg/dl are a warning, and the dose of the SU should be reduced. Conversely, once the fasting glucose concentrations are consistently at goal levels, before-supper values >200 mg/dl often predict that bedtime insulin with daytime oral antidiabetes drugs will not result in acceptable diabetes control. This decision is usually made, however, when an A1C level is obtained 3 months after the FPG target is achieved. If that value is >7.5% (rather than 7.0% for reasons discussed above), either a glitazone can be added or the SU can be discontinued, and the patient given two or more injections of insulin (see Regimens of Multiple Insulin Injections). The SU is stopped at this point because β-cell function is too low to control glycemia during the day and therefore would add little to two or more injections of insulin. Metformin is continued in obese/overweight patients to control weight gain but can be discontinued in lean patients. If a glitazone is added, simply use the maximal dose for reasons discussed previously and measure an A1C level 3 months later. Before-supper measurements of glucose levels are helpful to avoid hypoglycemia from the SU (see above) should the added glitazone be effective.

When should bedtime insulin plus daytime oral antidiabetes drugs be judged ineffective and a multiple-dose insulin regimen be instituted? A multiple-dose insulin regimen should not be instituted until the goal fasting glucose concentrations are achieved and A1C levels 3 months later are too high. A common error is to give up before reaching goal fasting glucose concentrations. This usually occurs in obese patients in whom not enough insulin is prescribed and the fasting glucose levels hover around the mid to high 100s. Sometimes over 100 units of insulin at bedtime must be prescribed to achieve the desired fasting range of glucose concentrations. Overnight hypoglycemia is seldom a problem because, as just mentioned, the insulin doses are gradually increased, NPH insulin peaks around breakfast time (not in the middle of the night when given before supper), glargine and detemir insulins are peakless, and patients are strongly encouraged to eat a small bedtime snack. As with the decision to add bedtime insulin, an A1C level >7.5% is also used to signal the need to switch to a multiple-dose insulin regimen. Not only are multiple-dose insulin regimens much more difficult for patients if followed appropriately (there is more frequent SMBG required, more risk of hypoglycemia, especially during the daytime, and less flexibility with dietary and exercise patterns), but importantly, the microvascular complications (retinopathy and nephropathy) were markedly increased over a 4- to 9-year period at A1C levels >8%, but only slightly so with values between 7 and 8% (and rarely at A1C levels below 7%), as mentioned above (17–21).

REGIMENS OF MULTIPLE INSULIN INJECTIONS

An approximate time course of action of various insulin preparations is shown in Table 9.

Table 9. Time Course of Action of Different Insulins

Insulin	Description	Onset (h)	Peak (h)	Duration (h)
Lispro (Humalog)	Rapid-acting	0.25	1–2	3–4
Aspart (Novolog)	Rapid-acting	0.25	1–2	3–4

Insulin	Description	Onset (h)	Peak (h)	Duration (h)
Glulisine (Apidra)	Rapid-acting	0.25	1–2	3–4
Regular	Short-acting	0.5 to 1	2–4	4–6
NPH (Humulin, Novolin)	Intermediate-acting	3 to 4	8–14	20–24
Glargine (Lantus)	Peakless	Not applicable	Not applicable	24
Detemir (Levemir)	Peakless	Not applicable	Not applicable	~18

The relationship among insulin preparations, time of injection, maximal period of activity, and timing of test best reflecting insulin action are shown in Table 10.

Table 10. Relationship Between SMBG Test, Component of Insulin Prescription, and Time of Injection

Insulin	Time Injected	Period of Activity	Pre-prandial Test Best Reflecting Insulin Effect
Regular Lispro (Humolog) Aspart (Novolog) Glulisine (Apidra)	Before a meal	Between that meal and either the next one or bedtime (snack) if injected before supper	Before next meal or bedtime (snack) if injected before supper
NPH (Humulin, Novolin)	Before breakfast	Between lunch and supper	Before supper
NPH (Humulin, Novolin)	Before supper or bedtime	Overnight	Before breakfast
Glargine (Lantus) Detemir (Levemir)	Any time	24 h ~18 h	Before breakfast

Five preferred insulin regimens are shown in Table 11.

Table 11. Insulin Regimens

Regimen	Before Breakfast	Before Lunch	Before Supper	Before Bedtime
A	NPH/regular or rapid-acting	—	NPH/regular or rapid-acting	—
B	NPH/regular or rapid-acting	—	Regular or rapid-acting	NPH
C	Regular or rapid-acting	Regular or rapid-acting	NPH/regular or rapid-acting	
D	Regular or rapid-acting	Regular or rapid-acting	Regular or rapid-acting	NPH
E	Regular or rapid-acting	Regular or rapid-acting	Regular or rapid-acting	Glargine or detemir

Regular insulin should be injected 30 min before the designated meal, and the rapid-acting insulin should be injected at the beginning of the meal. Under certain circumstances (e.g., patients become hypoglycemic if rapid-acting insulin is injected at the beginning of the meal before enough carbohydrate is absorbed or if the amount of food to be eaten is uncertain), rapid-acting insulin can be injected just after the meal is completed. Evening NPH insulin in type 1 diabetic patients receiving preprandial rapid-acting insulin may not be a good choice compared with the peakless insulins because of the short duration of action of these rapid-acting insulins and the long period of time between meals, especially lunch and supper. With evening NPH insulin, there would be little coverage in the late afternoon between lunch and supper.

Because glargine and detemir are peakless insulins, they can be injected at any time. In a small minority, twice-daily injections may improve control compared with a single injection. It is more likely that detemir needs to be injected twice daily, especially in type 1 diabetic patients, because it may not last the entire 24 h. If the dose is split, equal amounts are given in each injection, since they are peakless, and fasting glucose concentrations are used to adjust both doses, which are changed in equal amounts.

Suggested initial doses for patients starting on insulin are shown in Table 12.

Table 12. Initial Insulin Doses

Regimen	Before Breakfast	Before Lunch	Before Supper	Before Bedtime
Overweight and Obese Subjects				
A	20 units NPH/4–6 units regular or rapid-acting insulin[a]	—	10 units NPH/4–6 units regular or rapid-acting insulin[b]	—
B	20 units NPH/4–6 units regular or rapid-acting insulin[a]	—	4–6 units regular or rapid-acting insulin[b]	10 units NPH insulin
C	6–8 units regular or rapid-acting insulin[a]	6–8 units regular or rapid-acting insulin	16 units NPH/6–8 units regular or rapid-acting insulin	
D	6–8 units regular or rapid-acting insulin[a]	6–8 units regular or rapid-acting insulin	6–8 units regular or rapid-acting insulin	16 units NPH insulin
E	6–8 units regular or rapid-acting insulin[a]	6–8 units regular or rapid-acting insulin	6–8 units regular or rapid-acting insulin	16 units glargine[c] or detemir[c] insulin
Lean Subjects				
A	10 units NPH/2–4 units regular or rapid-acting insulin[a]	—	6 units NPH/2–4 units regular or rapid-acting insulin[b]	—
B	10 units NPH/2–4 units regular or rapid-acting insulin[a]	—	2–4 units regular or rapid-acting insulin[b]	6 units NPH insulin
C	4 units regular or rapid-acting insulin[a]	4 units regular or rapid-acting insulin	10 units NPH/4 units regular or rapid-acting insulin	
D	4 units regular or rapid-acting insulin[a]	4 units regular or rapid-acting insulin	4 units regular or rapid-acting insulin	10 units NPH insulin
E	4 units regular or rapid-acting insulin[a]	4 units regular or rapid-acting insulin	4 units regular or rapid-acting insulin	10 units glargine[c] or detemir[c] insulin

[a]Increase only after the before-breakfast glucose concentration is consistently at target (usually 70–130 mg/dl) and the before-lunch glucose concentration is above target. [b]Increase only after the before-supper glucose concentration is consistently at target (usually 70–130 mg/dl) and the before-bedtime (snack) glucose concentration is above target. [c]Glargine and detemir are clear insulins (like the short- and rapid-acting insulins and unlike the cloudy intermediate-acting NPH insulin). They should not be mixed with other insulins because they may change the time course of action of the other clear insulins. Because they are peakless, they may be given at any time.

Adjustment of insulin doses. Establish a target range (the ADA recommends 70–130 mg/dl, unless there are special circumstances). If a test at a specific time of day (usually before a meal or the bedtime snack) is consistently too high or too low, raise or lower the appropriate insulin dose (as described below) by 10%, but no less than 2 units in lean patients or 4 units in overweight and obese patients. (See Chapter 2 for calculation of desirable body weight [DBW]; patients ≥120% of DBW are considered overweight or obese.) When dose adjustments are being made after first starting insulin, "too high" is defined as values exceeding the upper target level for 3 days in a row. Three days are used for patients receiving two or more insulin injections instead of the 2 days when first adjusting bedtime insulin added to oral antidiabetes drugs because of the added risk of daytime hypoglycemia. Be sure that an aberrant high glucose value doesn't inadvertently expose the patient to this risk.

After the dose is stabilized, glucose concentrations at a specific time are too high if the number of values that exceed the upper target level *minus* the number of values that are less than the lower target level (plus bona fide *unexplained* hypoglycemic reactions for which no measured low glucose level is available) constitute 50% or more of the glucose concentrations at that time of day during a 1- to 6-week period (e.g., ≥4/7, ≥5/10, ≥7/14, ≥11/21, ≥14/28, ≥18/35, ≥21/42, or ≥50% of the values at any time between 1 and 6 weeks).

Conversely, the glucose concentrations at a specific time are "too low" if the number of values that are less than the lower target level (plus bona fide *unexplained* hypoglycemic reactions for which no measured low glucose value is available) *minus* the number of values that exceed the upper target level constitute ≥50% of the glucose concentrations at that time of day during a 1- to 6-week period. If the glucose concentrations at a specific time of day are neither too high nor too low, no change is made in that component of the insulin prescription that primarily affects the test at that time of day.

If high or low individual values are identified by the patient as being secondary to an unusual lifestyle event (e.g., rebound hyperglycemia after hypoglycemia either documented by SMBG or not, a delayed or missed meal, a larger carbohydrate-containing meal than usual, an unanticipated change in the usual exercise pattern), those values are not included in the analysis. Be careful not to lead the patient to this explanation. Many are likely to agree, so they don't "disappoint" the provider. Ask as neutrally as you can.

For patients on stable doses of insulin and A1C levels <7.5%, review their SMBG values at least every 6 weeks. For patients less well controlled, more frequent review of their SMBG values is helpful.

The relationship between the SMBG test and which component of the insulin prescription to adjust in the various regimens is shown in Table 13.

Table 13. Relationship of SMBG Tests and Adjustments of Doses in Different Insulin Regimens

Test	Regimen	Component to Adjust
If before breakfast too high or too low	A, C	NPH before supper
	B, D	NPH before bedtime
	E	Glargine or detemir (whenever taken)
If before lunch too high or too low	A, B, C, D, E	Regular or rapid-acting before breakfast
If before supper too high or too low	A, B	NPH before breakfast
	C, D, E	Regular or rapid-acting before lunch
If before bedtime snack too high or too low	A, B, C, D, E	Regular or rapid-acting before supper

Caveats

Regimens A and B. These regimens are called "mixed/split" because the insulin preparations are mixed in the same syringe and injected more than once a day. If used properly, this approach can yield as tight control as a basal/bolus regimen (39,40). However, patients have the least flexibility with their eating (and exercise) patterns. The before-supper and before-breakfast glucose concentrations are brought down to 70–130 mg/dl with the appropriate NPH insulin doses before regular or rapid-acting insulin is increased. This is because larger doses of the short- or rapid-acting insulins will be necessary to lower the before-lunch and before-bedtime (snack) glucose concentrations to target ranges when the before-breakfast and before-supper values, respectively, are higher than when they are lower. For example, to reach a before-lunch glucose concentration of <130 mg/dl will require more regular insulin when the fasting glucose concentration is 250 mg/dl than when it is 120 mg/dl. Delaying the increase of the short-acting insulin until the doses of NPH insulin have started to achieve better control reduces the possibility of hypoglycemic reactions.

Another approach to eventually getting the patient on a mixed/split regimen is to start with twice-daily NPH insulin and add regular or rapid-acting insulin *only* when the fasting and pre-supper glucose concentrations reach target values. For several reasons, this approach is not preferred. Almost all patients who require insulin will not achieve target A1C levels without regular or rapid-acting insulin. In my experience, there is often a great delay in starting the regular or rapid-acting insulin when the fasting and before-supper targets are reached. Moreover, often fasting and pre-supper glucose concentrations do not reach target at the same time, so that one has to start regular or rapid-acting insulin before the appropriate meal at two separate times, further complicating starting the short- or rapid-acting insulins.

Therefore, as shown in Table 12, include a small amount of regular or rapid-acting insulin initially, but wait until the before-breakfast and before-supper target glucose values are reached (or nearly so) before adjusting them further. Initially, patients only need to test before breakfast and before supper for adjustments of the NPH insulin doses. Since most patients will not test four times a day, once target glucose values are reached 50% or more of the time before breakfast or supper, patients are asked to start alternate testing, i.e., before breakfast and before lunch (when breakfast targets are reached) and before supper and before the bedtime snack (when supper targets are reached). (As stated above, all patients on insulin should have a small bedtime snack to avoid overnight hypoglycemia.) Hence, necessary information for adjusting doses for all components of the insulin prescription is gathered, although it takes twice as long to obtain it compared with testing four times a day. From a practical point of view, it is often better to start with NPH alone for several weeks, so that the patient can get used to injecting insulin and testing before introducing the mixing of insulins.

Given that the peak effect of NPH insulin taken before supper occurs between 8 and 14 h later, as this dose is increased to control the FPG concentration, hypoglycemia may occur overnight before the target is reached. Decreasing the before-supper dose may well avoid the overnight hypoglycemia but will work against achieving the fasting goal. If the patient is already taking a bedtime snack, that option is not available to avoid the overnight hypoglycemia. In that event, moving the NPH insulin to bedtime will almost always take care of the problem because the peak effect of the evening intermediate-acting insulin is now just before breakfast when the patient is about to eat. This converts the two-injection mixed/split regimen to a three-injection regimen. However, it is often the only way to both avoid overnight hypoglycemia and meet the fasting glycemia target without converting to a basal/bolus four-injection regimen.

Regimens C and D. These regimens are called "basal/bolus." Note that this term includes only the approach that uses the NPH insulin in the evening to control the FPG concentration. If NPH insulin is also given in the morning, the approach would be a mixed/split one with an additional injection of a short-acting insulin before lunch. This latter approach is not recommended because the before-supper glucose concentration is affected by both the morning NPH insulin and the short-acting insulin before lunch. Therefore, it is not clear which insulin dose should be adjusted. One caveat to the preprandial regular or rapid-acting/NPH basal/bolus regimen is that if there is a long period of time between lunch and supper, the effect of the before-lunch insulin injection might wane, and patients would experience high before-supper glucose concentrations. This potential problem is much more likely if a rapid-acting insulin is the preprandial insulin preparation used. Type 1 diabetic patients, who have no endogenous insulin secretion, are more likely to experience this than type 2 diabetic patients, who do have some endogenous insulin secretion. Patients using a basal/bolus regimen have more flexibility in regard to the timing of their meals and exercise than those on a mixed/split regimen. This can be important for some patients.

Regimen E. This regimen is also a basal/bolus regimen, with glargine or detemir insulin providing the basal component. Although glargine and detemir are peakless insulins, a long period of time between lunch and supper in some type 1 diabetic patients may result in glucose levels that are too high before supper after the effect of the before-lunch regular or rapid-acting insulin wears off. A second injection of glargine or detemir in the morning may help this problem.

Mixture insulins. Premixed NPH/regular insulins are available as 70/30 (70% NPH/30% regular), 50/50 (50% NPH/50% regular), and 75/25 (75% NPH/25% lispro). Although they obviate the need to have patients mix two different insulin preparations in the same syringe before injection, they have a major drawback. *One cannot adjust the doses of the NPH and shorter-acting insulins separately.* For example, if a patient on a 70/30 preparation had high before-lunch glucose concentrations but acceptable or low before-supper values, raising the morning dose to lower the before-lunch levels would jeopardize the before-supper situation. Therefore, achieving near-euglycemia with mixture insulins is often not possible, and these insulin preparations should be used only by patients who cannot be taught to mix insulins themselves and for whom no family or other caregiver is available. In my experience, most patients can be taught to mix insulin with persistent instruction.

Single morning injection. If this regimen is used, near-euglycemia is seldom achieved. This approach requires that the single morning injection of NPH insulin control both the before-supper glucose concentration and the following morning's value. The usual scenario is that as the morning NPH insulin dose is raised, the before-supper glucose concentrations become acceptable before the fasting ones. As the NPH insulin dose is increased further to lower the before-breakfast concentrations, late-afternoon hypoglycemia occurs, and the morning NPH insulin dose must be stabilized or decreased before target fasting levels are reached. At this point, evening NPH insulin must be introduced to improve control further (i.e., the patient is now on a mixed/split regimen, which should have been the initial approach).

Delayed response to NPH insulin. An occasional patient has a delayed response to NPH insulin, i.e., the peak effect of a morning injection occurs overnight so that the next day's fasting glucose concentration is affected more than the before-supper value. In this very unusual situation, a single morning injection of NPH insulin is appropriate, with regular or rapid-acting insulin given preprandially as necessary. Interestingly, the response to shorter-acting insulins remains normal. This suggests that the reason for the delayed response involves a slowed release of insulin from the protamine in the NPH preparation rather than a general delay in the egress of insulin from the subcutaneous space into the circulation. Patients with a delayed response to NPH insulin are usually identified by recognizing that the FPG concentrations remain low as the evening NPH insulin dose in a mixed/split regimen continues to be reduced and remains normal or low even when no evening NPH insulin is injected. These patients can be challenging to control. The FPG concentration reflects the action of the previous morning's NPH insulin. That dose is changed according to the pattern of FPG values. Preprandial regular or rapid-acting insulin is then necessary to control glucose concentrations during the day. Fortunately, this delayed response to NPH insulin does not occur very often.

Correction (supplemental) doses. Assuming no change in the carbohydrate content of the usual meal, high preprandial glucose concentrations require additional short- or rapid-acting insulin to lower the subsequent preprandial SMBG value into the target range. Table 14 shows the extra doses of insulins to start with to add to (or subtract from) the usual doses to "correct" the elevated glucose concentrations.

To evaluate the responses to these corrections doses, use a target range for the subsequent preprandial SMBG value of 100–150 mg/dl. If the majority of responses to a specific correction dose is >150 mg/dl, the correction dose needs to be increased; if the majority is <100 mg/dl (plus episodes of undocumented hypoglycemia), it should be decreased. A minimum of three responses to a specific correction dose is necessary before it can be evaluated. For example, if there are five instances where the patient added 2 units of regular insulin for preprandial SMBG values between 201 and 250 mg/dl, and the subsequent preprandial results were >150 mg/dl on four occasions, the cor-

Table 14. Initial Correction (Supplemental) Doses of Short- or Rapid-Acting Insulin

Blood Glucose (mg/dl)	Lean[a]	Overweight/Obese[b]
<70	−1 unit	−2 units
70–150	0 units	0 units
151–200	+1 unit	+2 units
201–250	+2 units	+4 units
251–300	+3 units	+6 units
301–350	+4 units	+8 units
>350	+5 units	+10 units

[a]<120% of DBW as calculated in Chapter 2. [b]≥120% DBW as calculated in Chapter 2.

rection dose for this preprandial range would be increased to +3 units, so that this amount of short- or rapid-acting insulin would be added for the preprandial range of 201–300 mg/dl. If subsequent experience showed that this correction dose was inadequate for the preprandial range of 251–300 mg/dl, the correction dose should be increased to +4 units for this latter range of preprandial values. To simplify the evaluation, it is helpful if patients record the usual dose and the correction dose separately (e.g., 3 + 2) in a logbook before the meal.

There are two ways to decide on a usual dose of short- or rapid-acting insulin. More sophisticated patients can learn carbohydrate counting, and the entire pre-prandial dose of these insulins is based on the amount of carbohydrate to be ingested, usually 1 unit per 10 or 15 g (41). In a mixed/split regimen, this dose would work for breakfast and supper but would not be suitable for lunch. This is because, as mentioned previously, both the morning NPH insulin and the short- or rapid-acting insulin before lunch have their maximal effects between lunch and supper. It would not be clear which dose of insulin to adjust in response to the pre-supper SMBG values. It would also be a third injection of insulin for the patient, negating one of the advantages of the two-injection mixed/split regimen.

The other dietary approach is a constant carbohydrate one in which patients are instructed on the carbohydrate content of various meal products and asked to ingest a relatively consistent amount of carbohydrate at each meal, i.e., a similar amount at each breakfast, lunch, and supper from day to day (not the same amount at each meal during the day). There is no evidence that carbohydrate counting leads to better control than the constant carbohydrate dietary approach (which is similar to the older Exchange System)

(42). With this approach, the preprandial short- or rapid-acting insulin dose (in both a mixed/split or basal/bolus regimen) can be broken down into three components. The "basic dose" is the amount prescribed to be taken before the meal and is the dose adjusted based on the pattern of SMBG values as described above. The "correction (supplemental) dose" depends on the preprandial glucose concentration. Some patients are also able to incorporate an "anticipatory dose" that depends on anticipated activities to occur with the meal or in the several hours after it. For instance, if patients are eating at a Chinese restaurant, they may add a few units (in addition to any correction dose), anticipating a higher carbohydrate meal than usual. Alternatively, if patients are going to engage in more exercise than usual after supper, they may reduce the short- or rapid-acting insulin dose taken before the meal that would have been dictated by the basic and correction doses. There is no formula for anticipatory doses. They must be arrived at empirically based on the patients' ongoing experiences.

GLYCEMIA ALGORITHM

Drug choices are limited to those available in the Los Angeles County formulary. (Incretins are not available.)

1. Principles of treatment: Type 1 diabetic patients require insulin. Type 2 diabetes is a progressive disease. The initial treatment for these patients is medical nutrition therapy, increased physical activity, and metformin. Over time, combinations of different classes of oral drugs are subsequently required. Over more time, insulin is often necessary.
2. Goals:
   a) Fasting plasma glucose (FPG) concentration <130 mg/dl.
   b) A1C level <7% (in a DCCT-standardized assay with normal range of 4–6%). This is the most important goal.
3. Progression of treatment in type 2 diabetic patients:
   a) Diet and exercise should be used initially and continuously in conjunction with all therapies.
   b) Monotherapy: All type 2 diabetic patients should be started on metformin, 500 mg twice daily, with meals (unless contraindicated). Measure FPG concentration in 2–3 weeks. If value >130 mg/dl, increase by one step (500 mg). Continue to increase by one step every 2–3 weeks until either:

(1) FPG is ≤130 mg/dl (then wait 3 months and measure an A1C level), or

(2) Maximal (tolerated) dose is reached, and FPG is still >130 mg/dl. In that case, start a sulfonylurea agent, 10 mg glipizide, 5 mg glyburide, or 2 mg glimepiride. Glimepiride is preferred because it is taken only once per day, even at higher doses. Also, glyburide causes more hypoglycemia than glipizide or glimepiride.

c) Dual therapy: Continue to measure the FPG concentration every 2–3 weeks. Increase the sulfonylurea agent by one step (10 mg for glipizide, 5 mg for glyburide, or 2 mg for glimepiride) until either:

(1) FPG is ≤130 mg/dl; then wait 3 months and measure an A1C level), or

(2) Maximal dose of the sulfonylurea agent is reached (glipizide, 20 mg twice daily; glyburide, 10 mg twice daily, or glimepiride, 8 mg once daily) and FPG is still >130 mg/dl. Measure an A1C level, and if >7.0%, add a maximal dose of pioglitazone (45 mg).

(3) Equivalent doses (mg) of the three sulfonylurea agents are as follows:

Glimepiride	Glipizide	Glyburide
2	10	5
4	20	10
6	30	15
8*	40*	20*

*Maximal dose.

d) Triple therapy

(1) Since it takes at least 8 weeks to see a substantial effect and can take up to 12–16 weeks before a maximal effect of a glitazone is seen, a decision on its effectiveness is made 4 months after starting pioglitazone.

(2) If A1C is >7.5% 4 months later, start bedtime insulin and discontinue pioglitazone.

e) Bedtime insulin

(1) Start obese patients with 16 units of NPH insulin and lean patients with 10 units of NPH insulin at bedtime.

(2) Gradually increase insulin dose until SMBG values before breakfast are 70–130 mg/dl >50% of the time.

(3) Wait 3 months and measure an A1C level.

(4) If A1C is >7.5%, switch to mixed/split regimen (or basal/bolus regimen if patient eats very irregularly).

f) Two or more daily injections of insulin: Adjust each component of the insulin regimen until ≥50% of appropriate preprandial SMBG values are within target range (70–130 mg/dl).

g) Relationship of each component of the insulin regimen and SMBG test best reflecting its effect:

Insulin	Time Injected	Best Test Reflecting Insulin Action
Regular Lispro Aspart Glulisine	Before a meal	Both following meal before which insulin is injected and before next meal or bedtime snack (if insulin taken before supper)
NPH	Before breakfast	Before supper
NPH	Before supper or bedtime	Before breakfast
Glargine Detemir	Before breakfast or before supper or half of dose at each time	Before breakfast

4. Treatment of markedly symptomatic newly diagnosed type 2 diabetic patients

a) These patients have marked polyuria, polydipsia, and often blurring of vision and weight loss. Glucose concentrations frequently exceed 400 mg/dl. Almost all of these patients can be successfully treated with high doses of sulfonylurea agents.

(In the chart below, metformin is added to the maximal dose of the SU if not already started.)

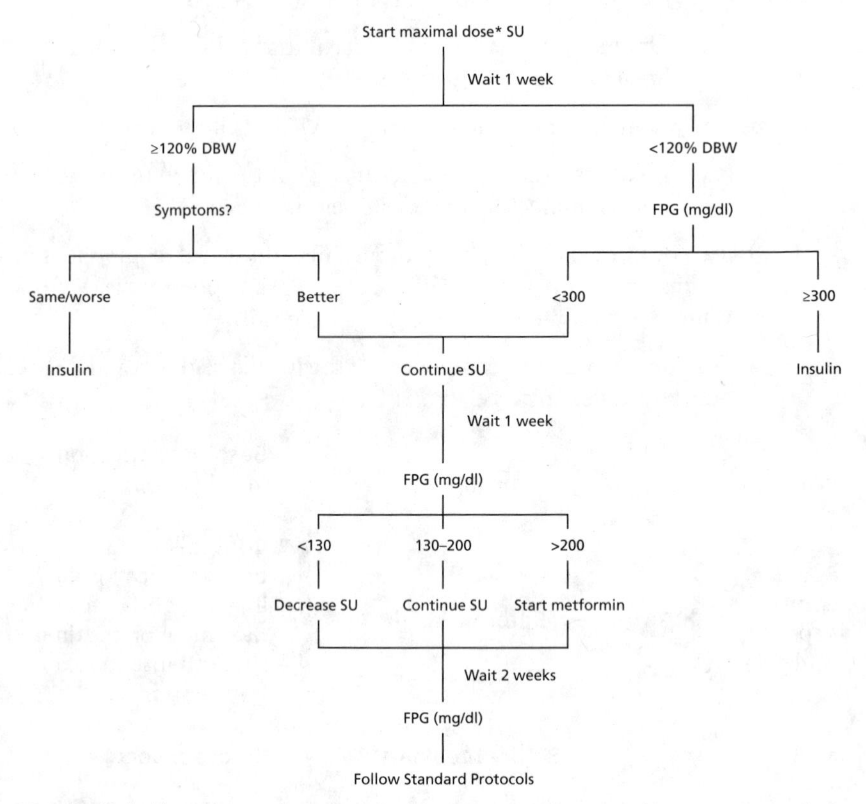

*Start with half-maximum dose if patient is >65 years of age, and increase to maximum dose at 1 week if no response.

References

1. Nathan DM, Buse JB, Davidson MB, Ferrannini E, Holman RR, Sherwin R, Zinman B: Medical management of hyperglycemia in type 2 diabetes: a consensus algorithm for the initiation and adjustment of therapy: a consensus statement from the American Diabetes Association and the European Association for the Study of Diabetes. *Diabetes Care* 32:193–203, 2009

2. Williams-Herman D, Round E, Swern AS, Musser B, Davies MJ, Stein PP, Kaufman KD, Amatruda JM: Safety and tolerability of sitagliptin in patients with type 2 diabetes: a pooled analysis. *BMC Endocrine Disorders* 8:14, 2008

3. Hermansen K, Kipnes M, Luo E, Fanurik D, Khatami H, Stein P: Efficacy and safety of the dipeptidyl-peptidase-4 inhibitor, sitagliptin, in patients with type 2 diabetes mellitus inadequately controlled on glimepiride alone or on glimepiride and metformin. *Diab Obes Metab* 9:733–745, 2007

4. Hsia SH, Navar MD, Duran P, Davidson MB: Non-inferiority of sitagliptin compared to thiazolidinediones as a third-line oral anti-hyperglycemic agent in ethnic minority type 2 diabetic patients: interim results. *Diabetes* 58 (Suppl. 1):A146, 2009

5. Heine RJ, Van Gaal LF, Johns D, Mihm MJ, Widel MH, Brodows, for the GWAA Study Group: Exenatide versus insulin glargine in patients with suboptimally controlled type 2 diabetes: a randomized trial. *Ann Intern Med* 143:559–569, 2005

6. Barnett AH, Burger J, Johns D, Brodows R, Kendall DM, Roberts A, Trautman ME: Tolerability and efficacy of exenatide and titrated insulin glargine in adult patients with type 2 diabetes previously uncontrolled with metformin or a sulfonylurea: a multinational, randomized, open label, two-period, crossover noninferiority trial. *Clin Ther* 29:2333–2348, 2007

7. Tran, MT, Navar MD, Davidson MB: Comparison of the glycemic effects of rosiglitazone and pioglitazone in triple oral therapy in type 2 diabetes mellitus. *Diabetes Care* 29:1395–1396, 2006

8. Aljabri K, Kozak SE, Thompson DM: Addition of pioglitazone or bedtime insulin to maximal doses of sulfonylurea and metformin in type 2 diabetes patients with poor glucose control: a prospective, randomized trial. *Am J Med* 116:230–235, 2004

9. Yki-Jarvinen H, Kauppila M, Kujansuu E, Lahti J, Marjanen T, Niskanen L, Rajala S, Ryysy L, Salo S, Seppala P, Tulokas T, Viikari J, Karjalainen J, Taskinen M-R: Comparison of insulin regimens in patients with non-insulin-dependent diabetes mellitus. *N Engl J Med* 327:1426–1433, 1992

10. Wolffenbuttal BH, Sets JP, Rondas-Colbers GJ, Menheere PP, Nieuwenhuijzen-Kruseman AC: Comparison of different regimens in elderly patients with NIDDM. *Diabetes Care* 19:1326–1332, 1996

11. Yki-Jarvinen H, Ryysy L, Kauppila M, Kujansuu E, Lahti J, Marjanen T, Niskanen L, Rajala S, Salo S, Seppala P, Tulokas T, Viikari J, Taskinen M-R: Effect of obesity on the response to insulin therapy in noninsulin-dependent diabetes mellitus. *J Clin Endocrinol Metab* 82:4037–4043, 1997

12. Yki-Jarvinen H, Ryysy L, Nikkila K, Tulokas T, Vanamo R, Heikkila M: Comparison of bedtime insulin in patients with type 2 diabetes mellitus: a randomized, controlled trial. *Ann Intern Med* 130:389–396, 1999

13. Kosaka K, Mizuno Y, Kuzuya T: Reproducibility of the oral glucose tolerance test and the rice-meal test in mild diabetics. *Diabetes* 15:901–904, 1966

14. Ollerton RL, Playle R, Ahmed K, Dunstan FD, Luzio SD, Owens DR: Day-to-day variability of fasting plasma glucose in newly diagnosed type 2 diabetic subjects. *Diabetes Care* 22:394–398, 1999

15. Nathan DM, Kuenen J, Borg R, Zheng H, Schoenfeld D, Heine RJ, for the A1C-Derived Glucose (ADAG) Study Group: Translating the A1C assay into estimated average glucose values. *Diabetes Care* 31:1473–1478, 2008

16. Shaw JS, Wilmot RL, Kilpatrick ES: Establishing pragmatic estimated GFR thresholds to guide metformin prescribing. *Diabet Med* 24:1160–1163, 2007

17. DCCT Research Group: The effect of intensive treatment of diabetes on the development of long-term complications in insulin-dependent diabetes mellitus. *N Engl J Med* 329:977–986, 1993

18. Krolewski AS, Laffel LMB, Krolewski M, Quinn M, Warram JH: Glycosylated hemoglobin and the risk of microalbuminuria in patients with insulin-dependent diabetes mellitus. *N Engl J Med* 332;1251–1255, 1995

19. Warram JH, Scott LJ, Hanna LS, Wantman M, Cohen SE, Laffel MB, Ryan L, Krolewski A: Progression of microalbuminuria to proteinuria in type 1 diabetes: nonlinear relationship with hyperglycemia. *Diabetes* 49:94–100, 2000

20. Ohkubo O, Kishikawa H, Araki E, Miyata T, Isami S, Motoyoshi S, Kojima Y, Furuyoshi N, Shichiri M: Intensive insulin therapy prevents the progression of diabetic microvascular complications in Japanese patients with noninsulin dependent mellitus: a randomized, prospective 6-year study. *Diabetes Res Clin Pract* 28:103–117, 1995

21. Tanaka Y, Atsumi Y, Matsuoka K, Onuma T, Tohjima T, Kawamori R: Role of glycemic control and blood pressure in the development and progression of nephropathy in elderly Japanese NIDDM patients. *Diabetes Care* 21:116–120, 1998

22. Heine RJ, Va Gael LF, Johns D, Mihm MJ, Widel MH, Brodows RG for the GWAA Group. Exenatide versus glargine in patients with suboptimally controlled type 2 diabetes: a randomized trial. *Ann Intern Med* 143:559-569, 2005

23. Schwartz AV, Selllmeyer DE, Vittinghoff E, Palermo L, Lecka-Czernik B, Feingold KR, Strotmeyer ES, Resnick HE, Carbonne L, Beamer BA, Park SW, Lane NE, Harris TB, Cummings SR: Thiazolidinedione use and bone loss in older diabetic adults. *J Clin Endocrinol Metab* 91:3349–3354, 2006

24. Grey A, Bolland M, Gamble G, Wattie D, Horne A, Davidson J, Reid IR: The peroxisome-proliferator-activated receptor-γ agonist rosiglitazone decreases bone formation and bone mineral density in healthy postmenopausal women: a randomized, controlled trial. *J Clin Endocrinol Metab* 92:1305–1310, 2007

25. Khan SE, Zinman B, Lachin JM, Haffner SM, Herman WH, Holman RR, Kravitz BG, Yu D, Heise MA, Aftring RP, Viberti G, for the A

Diabetes Outcome Progression Trial (ADOPT) Study Group. *Diabetes Care* 31:845–851, 2008

26. Meier C, Kraenzlin ME, Bodner M, Jick SS, Jick H, Meier CR: Use of thiazolidinediones and fracture risk. *Arch Intern Med* 168:820–825, 2008

27. Diamond GA, Bax L, Kaul S: Uncertain effects of rosiglitazone on the risk for myocardial infarction and cardiovascular death. *Ann Intern Med* 147:585–587, 2007

28. Nissen SE, Wolski K: Effect of rosiglitazone on the risk of myocardial infarction and death from cardiovascular causes. *N Engl J Med* 356:2457–2471, 2006

29. Singh S, Loke YK, Furberg CD: Long-term risk of cardiovascular events with rosiglitazone: a meta-analysis. *JAMA* 298:1189–1195, 2007

30. Home PD, Pocock SJ, Beck-Nielsen H, Curtis PS, Gomis R, Hanefeld M, Jones NP, Komajda M, McMurray JJV, for the RECORD Study Group: Rosiglitazone evaluated for cardiovascular outcomes in oral agent combination therapy for type 2 diabetes (RECORD): a multicentre, randomized, open-label trial. *Lancet* 373:2125–2135, 2009

31. Lincoff AM, Wolski K, Nicholls SJ, Nissen SE: Pioglitazone and risk of cardiovascular events in patients with type 2 diabetes mellitus: a meta-analysis of randomized trials. *JAMA* 298:1180–1188, 2007

32. Wilcox R, Kupfer S, Erdmann E, on behalf of the PROactive Study Investigators: Effects of pioglitazonoe on major adverse cardiovascular events in high-risk patients with type 2 diabetes: results from PROprospective pioglitAzone Clinical Trial In macro Vascular Events (PROactive 10). *Am Heart J* 155:712–717, 2008

33. Peters AL, Davidson MB: Maximal-dose glyburide in markedly symptomatic patients with type 2 diabetes: a new use for an old friend. *J Clin Endocrinol Metab* 81:2423–2427, 1996

34. Karter AJ, Ackerson LM, Darbinian JA, D'Agostino RB, Ferrara A, Liu J, Selby JV: Self-monitoring of blood glucose levels and glycemic control: the Northern California Kaiser Permanente Diabetes Registry. *Am J Med* 111:1–9, 2001

35. Davidson MB: Self monitoring of blood glucose in type 2 diabetic patients not receiving insulin: a waste of money. *Diabetes Care* 28:1531–1533, 2005

36. Davidson MB, Castellanos M, Duran P, Karlan V: Effective diabetes care by a registered nurse following treatment algorithms in a minority population. *Am J Manag Care* 12:226–232, 2006

37. Davidson MB: How our current medical care system fails people with diabetes: lack of timely, appropriate clinical decisions. *Diabetes Care* 32:370–372, 2009

38. Hsia S: Single-dose regimens of insulin glargine compared to NPH in ethnic minority type 2 diabetic patients uncontrolled on oral agents: interim results. *Diabetes* 57 (Suppl. 1):A60, 2008

39. Reeves ML, Seigler DE, Ryan EA, Skyler JS: Glycemic control in insulin-dependent diabetes mellitus: comparison of outpatient intensified conventional therapy with continuous subcutaneous insulin infusion. *Am J Med* 72:673–680, 1982

40. Umpierrez GE, Hor T, Smiley D, Temponi A, Umpierrez D, Ceron M, Munoz C, Newton C, Peng L, Baldwin D: Comparison of inpatient insulin regimens with detemir plus aspart *versus* neutral protamne Hagedorn plus regular in medical patients with type 2 diabetes. *J Clin Endocrinol Metab* 94:564–569, 2009

41. Kulkarni K: Carbohydrate counting for pump therapy. In *A Core Curriculum for Diabetes Education: Diabetes Management Therapies.* 5th ed. Franz MJ, Ed. American Association of Diabetes Educators, Chicago, IL. 265–276, 2003

42. American Diabetes Association: Nutrition recommendations and interventions for diabetes (Position Statement). *Diabetes Care* 29:2140–2157, 2006

43. Schutt SM, Kern W, Krause U, Busch P, Dapp A, Grziwotz R, Mayer I, Rosenbauer J, Wagner C, Zimmermann A, Kerner W, Holl RW: DPV Initiative: Is the frequency of self-monitoring of blood glucose related to long-term metabolic control? Multicenter analysis including 24,500 patients from 191 centers in Germany and Austria. *Exp Clin Endocrinol Diabetes* 114:384–388, 2006

Chapter 4 Dyslipidemia

GOALS OF THERAPY

As discussed in Chapter 1, macrovascular disease is much more common in people with diabetes than their counterparts without diabetes. Coronary artery disease (CAD) is twice as common in men with diabetes and four to five times more common in women with diabetes. Lowering low density lipoprotein (LDL) cholesterol levels in people with diabetes reduces their risk of CAD, as it does in those without diabetes (1). In fact, the cardiovascular events and mortality in diabetic patients with elevated LDL cholesterol levels taking a statin were almost equivalent to a comparable nondiabetic population not receiving a statin (2). Furthermore, studies that included patients with and without diabetes have demonstrated some regression of lesions in the coronary arteries when the LDL cholesterol levels are lowered to <100 mg/dl (3).

The situation regarding triglyceride (TG) levels is not as straightforward. Although many studies have shown an association between elevated TG levels and CAD (4), the fact that low high density lipoprotein (HDL) levels (also a risk factor for CAD) are associated with elevated TG levels obscures this relationship. Intervention studies (i.e., tracking outcomes in populations given TG-lowering agents or a placebo) have not shown clear-cut results. In the Helsinki Heart Study (5), gemfibrozil, a fibrate that lowers TG levels, significantly decreased cardiac end points in men with primary dyslipidemia. However, LDL cholesterol levels were also decreased, and HDL cholesterol levels were increased. The importance of the latter was underscored by the Veterans Affairs High-Density Lipoprotein Intervention Trial (VA-HIT) study (6), a secondary prevention study in which men with low HDL cholesterol levels and normal LDL cholesterol and TG levels were recruited. As expected, gemfibrozil raised HDL cholesterol levels, which were inversely related to CAD events. In a recent report on a large number of patients with type 2 diabetes, the FIELD study (7), the overall cardiovascular disease (CVD) event rate was not reduced by fenofibrate (another fibrate). A significant decrease of non-fatal myocardial infarctions was counterbalanced by a significant increase of fatal ones. However, there are some indirect data to strongly suggest that lowering TG levels may be beneficial for people with CAD. In the presence of high TG levels, the LDL particle becomes smaller and denser. This altered lipoprotein particle is more atherogenic in vitro, and in prospective studies it predicts myocardial infarctions.

Three studies (8–10) have shown that the presence of diabetes in patients without a previous myocardial infarction imposes the same risk of death from CAD as does a previous myocardial infarction in patients without diabetes. Based on these data, the third report of the National Cholesterol Education Program (NCEP) Expert Panel on Detection, Evaluation, and Treatment of High Blood Cholesterol in Adults (Adult Treatment Panel III), known as ATP III (11), recommended that the goal for LDL cholesterol levels in people with diabetes and no clinical evidence of CAD be <100 mg/dl. If clinical evidence is present, the goal should be <70 mg/dl.

In contrast to individual studies in which TG levels could not be clearly implicated as an independent risk factor for CAD, the ATP III report (11) states that recent meta-analyses of prospective studies do show that elevated TG levels are an independent risk factor. This suggests that some TG-rich lipoproteins, called remnant lipoproteins, are atherogenic. A surrogate measure of remnant lipoproteins is non-HDL cholesterol, which is simply calculated as total cholesterol minus HDL cholesterol. Therefore, after an LDL cholesterol concentration of <100 mg/dl (or <70 mg/dl) is achieved, attention should be directed to TG concentrations. If these concentrations are ≥200 mg/dl, the non-HDL cholesterol level should be calculated. If that value is >30 mg/dl above the LDL cholesterol goal, further treatment should be instituted to meet the non-HDL cholesterol target. This should be to increase the statin dose, and if a maximal dose of atorvastatin or rosuvastatin is reached, ezetimibe should be added (see below). If the non-HDL cholesterol target is still not met, adding fenofibrate can be considered. However, it is recommended to only add the fibrate if the non-HDL cholesterol at that point is ≥160 mg/dl because of the increased chances of side effects with both a statin and a fibrate and the fact that a meta-analysis of four large studies showed that the increase in CAD mortality only occurred at levels ≥160 mg/dl (not 130–159 mg/dl) in people with and without diabetes (12).

PRINCIPLES OF TREATMENT

All diabetic patients ≥40 years of age should be started on a statin regardless of the baseline LDL cholesterol level. The reason is that statins have beneficial effects on CVD, independent of their ability to lower cholesterol levels (13). Statin therapy should also be considered in patients <40 years old with multiple CVD risk factors if the LDL cholesterol levels remain ≥100 mg/dl after lifestyle modification, i.e., reduction of dietary saturated and trans fats, weight loss (if indicated), and increased physical activity.

The initial statin dose should be increased monthly until the goal cholesterol level is achieved. If the maximal dose of a generic statin does not achieve goal levels, the patient should be switched to the maximal dose of a more effective statin, atorvastatin (soon to be generic) or rosuvastatin. If one of these statins does not achieve this target level, ezetimibe (an inhibitor of cholesterol absorption from the gastrointestinal [GI] tract) should be added. Alternatively, for cost considerations, ezetimibe can be added to the maximal dose of a generic statin, and if this combination fails to achieve goal levels, atorvastatin or rosuvastatin can be substituted for the generic statin. If the combination of maximal doses of atorvastatin or rosuvastatin plus ezetimibe is inadequate, the addition of a niacin preparation or a bile acid resin could be considered, especially if the patient is at very high risk. Note that niacin preparations also effectively lower TG levels, whereas bile acid resins increase them somewhat. Alternatively, if the absolute LDL cholesterol targets cannot be reached, the ADA guidelines are to reduce the baseline values by at least 30–40%.

TG levels ≥1,000 mg/dl can cause pancreatitis and should be treated initially with fenofibrate in addition to a statin.

The approach to documenting dyslipidemia depends on whether the LDL cholesterol level can be measured directly or can only be calculated from the following equation:

LDL cholesterol = total cholesterol – HDL cholesterol – TG/5

If the TG level is >400 mg/dl, the calculated LDL cholesterol concentration is inaccurate. In that case, a fibrate is used to reduce TG levels to <400 mg/dl, so that LDL cholesterol concentrations can be calculated. Fenofibrate should be the fibrate used because there are fewer side effects when added to a statin compared with gemfibrozil. When the TG concentration decreases to <400 mg/dl and LDL cholesterol can be more accurately calculated, fenofibrate is discontinued. If the TG level remains >400 mg/dl, fenofibrate is continued and the non-HDL cholesterol level is used to adjust the statin dose with a goal of 30 mg/dl above the usual statin goal for that patient. If the TG level has fallen to <400 mg/dl on fenofibrate but increased to above that value when the fibrate is discontinued, it should be added back so that LDL cholesterol levels can be followed.

If direct measurements of LDL cholesterol concentrations are available, elevated values can be treated regardless of the TG level. The two approaches (of whether direct LDL cholesterol measurements are available or not) are described in the Dyslipidemia Algorithm below.

Omega-3 polyunsaturated fatty acids (PUFAs) (or fish oils) will lower triglyceride levels without much effect on HDL cholesterol levels. LDL cholesterol levels may increase modestly, but the particle that carries LDL cholesterol changes from the more atherogenic, smaller, denser size to one that is larger, more buoyant (less dense), and less atherogenic. A systematic review (which noted the possibility of publication bias whereby neutral or negative trials may not be published) showed that supplementation with fish oils was associated with a significant reduction in deaths due to cardiac causes and no effect on arrhythmias or all-cause mortality (14). The PUFA content of fish oil preparations in health food stores is variable. A highly concentrated PUFA preparation, Lovaza (formerly called Omacor), is approved by the Food and Drug Administration as an adjunct to diet for the treatment of very high triglyceride levels (>500 mg/dl).

ADVERSE EVENTS

In general, adverse events due to medications for dyslipidemia are uncommon. With statins, the most common adverse event is myalgias, which rarely progresses to rhabdomyolysis, which can cause renal failure. Adverse effects occur in ~0.2% of patients taking a statin alone, <5% of patients on a combination of a fibrate and a statin, and up to 30% of patients on this combined therapy with the addition of erythromycin or cyclosporine. Periodic monitoring of patients on a combination of a statin and a fibrate with creatinine phosphokinase (CPK) levels is appropriate. The combination should be discontinued if the levels exceed 5–10 times normal. Periodic monitoring of hepatic transaminases is appropriate with the combination of fibrates and statins (although not necessarily with either alone). As stated above, if used in combination, fenofibrate is preferred over gemfibrozil because of lower chances of side effects. The offending drug(s) should be discontinued if the level of either of these two hepatic enzymes (ALT, AST) exceed three times normal. A fibrate also can cause GI disturbances.

Niacin commonly causes flushing, pruritus, and GI upset after ingestion, although these are less frequent with the extended-release preparations. These side effects gradually subside on continued usage. Because they are prostaglandin mediated, aspirin 30 min before taking niacin will lessen the cutaneous symptoms. Niacin can also cause hepatotoxicity and hyperuricemia, and higher doses increase insulin resistance leading to deterioration of glucose control.

Bile acid binding resins can cause bloating and constipation and may interfere with absorption of other drugs. This is less common with colesevelam, the newest preparation. A potential added advantage with colesevelam is that the drug lowers A1C levels by ~0.5% compared with a placebo (15,16). Bile acid binding resins often increase triglyceride levels.

PUFAs are generally well tolerated. Side effects include eructation, dyspepsia, and perversion of taste. Diabetes control can also worsen, and they can inhibit platelet aggregation and may cause bleeding.

MEDICATIONS

Table 15 shows various generic and brand name drugs and their appropriate doses.

Table 15. Suggested Dosing Regimens for Drugs to Treat Dyslipidemia

Generic Name	Brand Name (tablet size)	Starting Dose	Dose Changes	Maximal Dose
Statins				
Lovastatin	Mevacor (10, 20, 40 mg)	20 mg QHS	By 20 mg (40 mg split to BID)	40 mg BID
	Altoprev (20, 40, 60 mg, extended-release tablet)	20 mg	By 20 mg	60 mg
Pravastatin	Pravachol (10, 20, 40, 80 mg)	10 mg QHS	Double each dose	80 mg QHS
Simvastatin	Zocor (5, 10, 20, 40, 80 mg)	10 mg QHS	Double each dose	80 mg QHS
Fluvastatin	Lescol (20, 40 mg)	20 mg QHS	By 20 mg (>40 mg, split to BID)	40 mg BID
	Lescol XL (80 mg, extended-release tablet)	80 mg	NA	80 mg
Atorvastatin[a]	Lipitor (10, 20, 40, 80 mg)	10 mg QD	Double each dose	80 mg QD
Rosuvastatin[a]	Crestor (5, 10, 20, 40 mg)	10 mg QD[b]	Double each dose	40 mg QD
Cholesterol Absorption Inhibitor				
Ezetimibe	Zetia	10 mg	Not applicable	10 mg
Bile Acid Binding Resins				
Cholestyramine	Questran (5 g per packet)	1 packet QD or BID	1 packet/ month	6 packets/ day

Generic Name	Brand Name (tablet size)	Starting Dose	Dose Changes	Maximal Dose
Colestipol	Colestid (5 g per packet)	1 packet QD or BID	1 packet/ month	6 packets/ day
Colesvelam[c]	Welchol (625 mg)	3 tablets twice a day with meals or 2 tablets three times a day with meals	Can add one extra table per day for a total of 7	7 tablets per day
Fibrates				
Gemfibrozil	Lopid (600 mg)	600 mg BID	Not applicable	600 mg BID
Fenofibrate[d]	Tricor (48, 145 mg)	48–145 mg QD	48 mg QD	145 mg QD
	Lofibra (67, 200 mg)	67–200 mg QD	67 mg QD	200 mg QD
	Generics (generics available in different strengths)	Lowest to highest tablet size of generic	By lowest dose of generic	Maximal tablet size of generic
Anti-Lipolytic				
Niacin	Generic (50, 100, 250, 500 mg)	100 mg before each meal for 2 weeks; 250 mg before each meal for 2 weeks	500 mg before each meal for 1 month, then 500-mg increase per month if necessary	4 g or maximally tolerated dose if less
Niacin ER (extended release)	Niaspan, Slo-Niacin (500, 750, 1,000 mg)	500 mg QHS	500 mg QHS per month as necessary	2 g QHS
Omega-3 PUFAs				
PUFA (ethyl esters of eicosapentaenoic acid [465 mg] and docosahexaenoic acid [375 mg])	Lovaza (1 g)	2 g BID or 4 g QD	Not applicable	4 g

Generic Name	Brand Name (tablet size)	Starting Dose	Dose Changes	Maximal Dose
Combination Drugs				
Vytorin (ezetimibe/simvastatin): 10/10, 10/20, 10/40, 10/80				
Advicor (niacin/lovastatin): 500/20, 750/20, 1,000/20				
Simcor (niacin/simvastatin): 500/20, 750/20, 1,000/20				

QHS – at hour of sleep (bedtime); QD – once per day; BID – twice per day

[a]Also lowers TG levels; can be taken at any time because of its long duration of action. [b]Start with 5 mg in patients with severe renal insufficiency (<30 ml/min) or subjects taking cyclosporine. [c]Less GI side effects than with the other bile acid binding resins; also ~0.5% A1C decrease. [d]Take with food. Start with 54 mg in elderly patients and any patient with impaired renal function. However, Los Angeles County only has a 130-mg generic formulation.

DYSLIPIDEMIA ALGORITHM

Drug choices are limited to those available in the Los Angeles County formulary.

TREATMENT PLAN (DIRECT LDL CHOLESTEROL MEASUREMENTS AVAILABLE)

1. Measure fasting baseline lipid panel. (Hepatic transaminases should be measured every time lipids are.)
2. All diabetic patients ≥40 years old should be taking a statin regardless of baseline LDL cholesterol concentration.
3. Goal level of LDL cholesterol is <100 mg/dl, or <70 mg/dl if patient has overt CVD.
4. Start a statin in all patients ≥40 years old, and consider it in patients <40 years old whose LDL cholesterol remains above goal levels after lifestyle modification or who have multiple CVD risk factors.
5. In patients not at goal level, measure LDL cholesterol 1 month after starting a statin; measure LDL cholesterol at monthly intervals, and increase dose of drug until goal level is achieved.
6. Drug titration.
   a) Start simvastatin (Zocor), 10 mg QHS, and double each month as follows until goal achieved; 10 mg → 20 mg → 40 mg → 80 mg; if goal still not achieved, switch to 80 mg atorvastatin (Lipitor); if goal

still not met 1 month later, add 10 mg ezetimibe (Zetia); if goal still not met 1 month later, CONSULT MD.

OR

b) Start Vytorin (combination of ezetimibe [Zetia] plus simvastatin) 10/10 mg QHS and increase each month as follows until goal achieved; 10/10 mg → 10/20 mg → 10/40 mg → 80 mg atorvastatin plus 10 mg ezetimibe (Los Angeles County formulary does not carry 10/80 of Vytorin); if goal not met 1 month later, CONSULT MD.

7. If initial TG concentration is ≥1,000 mg/dl, also start fenofibrate at 130 mg QD (generic tablet size available in the Los Angeles County formulary): measure TG concentration in 1 month.
   a) If TG concentration remains ≥1,000 mg/dl, continue fenofibrate and CONSULT MD.
   b) If TG concentration <1,000 mg/dl, discontinue fenofibrate but restart if subsequent TG concentrations increase to ≥1,000 mg/dl and CONSULT MD.
8. When LDL cholesterol is at goal, if TG concentration is 200–999 mg/dl, calculate the non-HDL cholesterol (non-HDL cholesterol = total cholesterol – LDL cholesterol); if this value is >130 mg/dl (>100 mg/dl in patients with overt CVD), keep increasing the statin dose (see 6a or 6b above) monthly until appropriate goal is reached.
9. If the patient reaches 80 mg atorvastatin plus 10 mg ezetimibe, and the non-HDL cholesterol value is 130–159 mg/dl, simply follow the patient; if the non-HDL cholesterol value is ≥160 mg/dl (and the patient is not taking fenofibrate), add 130 mg fenofibrate.
10. When LDL cholesterol (and non-HDL cholesterol if TG concentrations are 200–999 mg/dl) is at goal, measure lipids every 4 months during the subsequent year and every 6 months thereafter. Intensify treatment as described above if lipids increase above goal levels.

TREATMENT PLAN (DIRECT LDL CHOLESTEROL MEASUREMENTS NOT AVAILABLE)

1. Measure fasting baseline lipid panel. (Hepatic transaminases should be measured every time lipids are.)
2. All diabetic patients ≥40 years old should be taking a statin regardless of baseline LDL cholesterol concentration.
3. Goal level of LDL cholesterol is <100 mg/dl, or <70 mg/dl if patient has overt CVD.
4. Start a statin in all patients ≥40 years old, and consider it in patients <40

years old whose LDL cholesterol remains above goal levels after lifestyle modification or who have multiple CVD risk factors.

5. If initial TG concentration is <400 mg/dl and patient is not at LDL cholesterol goal level, measure LDL cholesterol 1 month after starting a statin; measure LDL cholesterol at monthly intervals, and increase dose of drug until goal level is achieved.
6. Drug titration.
   a) Start simvastatin (Zocor), 10 mg QHS, and double each month as follows until goal is achieved; 10 mg → 20 mg → 40 mg → 80 mg; if goal is still not achieved, switch to 80 mg atorvastatin (Lipitor); if goal still not met 1 month later, add 10 mg ezetimibe (Zetia); if goal still not met 1 month later, CONSULT MD.

   OR

   b) Start Vytorin (combination of ezetimibe [Zetia] plus simvastatin) 10/10 mg QHS and increase each month as follows until goal achieved; 10/10 mg → 10/20 mg → 10/40 mg → 80 mg atorvastatin plus 10 mg ezetimibe (Los Angeles County does not carry 10/80 of Vytorin); if goal not met 1 month later, CONSULT MD.
7. When LDL cholesterol is at goal level, if TG concentration is 200–399 mg/dl, calculate the non-HDL cholesterol (non-HDL cholesterol = total cholesterol – LDL cholesterol); if this value >130 mg/dl (>100 mg/dl in patients with overt CVD), keep increasing the statin dose (see 6a or 6b above) monthly until this goal is reached.
8. If the patient reaches 80 mg atorvastatin plus 10 mg ezetimibe, and the non-HDL cholesterol value is 130–159 mg/dl, simply follow the patient; if the non-HDL cholesterol value is ≥160 mg/dl (and the patient is not taking fenofibrate), add 130 mg fenofibrate.
9. If initial TG concentration is 400–999 mg/dl, calculate the non-HDL cholesterol; if this value is >130 mg/dl (>100 mg/dl in patients with overt CVD), keep increasing the statin dose (see 6a or 6b above) monthly until the appropriate goal is reached.
10. If the patient reaches 80 mg atorvastatin plus 10 mg ezetimibe and the non-HDL cholesterol value is 130–159 mg/dl, simply follow the patient; if the non-HDL cholesterol value is ≥160 mg/dl (and the patient is not taking fenofibrate), add 130 mg fenofibrate.
11. If initial TG concentration is ≥1,000 mg/dl, also start fenofibrate at 130 mg QD (generic tablet size available in the Los Angeles County formulary), along with 10 mg simvastatin QHS; measure TG concentration in 1 month.
    a) If TG concentration remains ≥1,000 mg/dl, continue fenofibrate and CONSULT MD.

b) If TG concentration is <1,000 mg/dl, discontinue fenofibrate, but restart it if subsequent TG concentrations increase to ≥1,000 mg/dl and CONSULT MD. If TG levels remain ≥400 mg/dl, use non-HDL cholesterol levels to adjust lipid medications.

12. When LDL cholesterol (and/or non-HDL cholesterol if TG concentrations are 200–999 mg/dl) is at goal, measure lipids every 4 months during the subsequent year and every 6 months thereafter. Intensify treatment as described above if lipids increase above goal levels.

References

1. Cholesterol Treatment Trialists' (CTT) Collaborators: Efficacy and safety of cholesterol-lowering treatment: prospective meta-analysis of data from 90,056 participants in 14 randomized trials of statins. *Lancet* 366:1267–1278, 2005

2. Sacks FM, Pfeffer MA, Moye LA, Rouleau JL, Rutherford JD, Cole TG, Brown L, Warnica JW, Arnold JM, Wunn CC, Davis BR, Braunwald E: The effect of pravastatin on coronary events after myocardial infarction in patients with average cholesterol levels. *N Engl J Med* 335:1001–1009, 1996

3. Nichols SJ, Tuzcu EM, Sipahi I, Grasso AW, Schoenhagen P, Hu T, Wolski K, Crowe T, Desai MY, Hazen SL, Kapadia SR, Nissen SE: Statins, high-density lipoprotein cholesterol, and regression of coronary atherosclerosis. *JAMA* 297:499–508, 2007

4. Sarwar N, Danesh J, Eriksdottir G, Sigurdsson G, Wareham N, Bingham S, Boekholdt SM, Khaw KT, Gudnason V: Triglycerides and the risk of coronary heart disease: 10,158 incident cases among 262,525 participants in 29 Western prospective studies. *Circulation* 115:450–458, 2007

5. Frick MH, Elo O, Haapa K, Heinsalmi P, Helo P, Huttunen JK, Kaitaniemi P: Helsinki Heart Study: primary-prevention trial with gemfibrozil in middle-aged men with dyslipidemia: safety of treatment, changes in risk factors, and incidence of coronary heart disease. *N Engl J Med* 317:1237–1245, 1987

6. Robins SJ, Collins D, Wittes JT, Papademetriou V, Deedwania PC, Schaefer EJ, McNamara JR, Kashyap ML, Hershman JM, Wexler JM, Rubins HB: VA-HIT Study Group, Veterans Affairs High-Density Lipoprotein Intervention Trial: Relation of gemfibrozil treatment and lipid levels with major coronary events: VA-HIT: a randomized controlled trial. *JAMA* 285:1585–1591, 2001

7. FIELD Investigators: Effects of long-term fenofibrate therapy on cardiovascular events in 9,795 people with type 2 diabetes mellitus (the FIELD study): randomized control trial. *Lancet* 366:1849–1861, 2005

8. Haffner SM, Lehto S, Ronnemaa T, Pyorala K, Laakso M: Mortality from coronary heart disease in subjects with type 2 diabetes and in non-diabetic subjects with and without prior myocardial infarction. *N Engl J Med* 339:229–234, 1998

9. Malmberg K, Yusuf S, Gerstein HC, Brown J, Zhao F, Hunt D, Piegas L, Calvin J, Keltai M, Budaj A: Impact of diabetes on long-term prognosis in patients with unstable angina and non-Q-wave myocardial infraction. *Circulation* 102:1014–1019, 2000

10. Muramal KJ, Nesto RW, Cohen MC, Muller JF, Maclure M, Sherwood JB, Mittleman MA: Impact of diabetes on long-term survival after acute myocardial infarction: comparability of risk with prior myocardial infarction. *Diabetes Care* 24:1422–1427, 2001

11. Grundy SM, Cleeman JI, Merz CN, Brewer HB Jr, Clark LT, Hunninghake DB, Pasternak RC, Smith SC Jr, Stone NJ: Implications of recent clinical trials for the National Cholesterol Education Program Adult Treatment Panel III guidelines. *Circulation* 110:227–239, 2004

12. Liu JL, Sempos C, Donahue RP, Dorn JD Trevisan M, Grundy SM: Joint distribution of non-HDL and LDL cholesterol and coronary heart disease risk prediction among individuals with and without diabetes. *Diabetes Care* 28:1916–1921, 2005

13. Paraslevas KI, Stathopoulas V, Mikhailidis DP: Pleiotropic effects of statins: implications for a wide range of diseases. *Curr Vasc Pharmacol* 6:237–239, 2008

14. Leon H, Shibata MC, Sivakumaran S, Dorgan M, Chatterly T, Tsuyuki RT: Effect of fish oil on arrythmias and mortality: systematic review. *BMJ* 338:a2931, 2008

15. Zieve FJ, Schwartz SL, Jones MR, Bailey WL: Results of the glucose-lowering effect of WelChol (GLOWS): a randomized, double-blind, placebo-controlled pilot study evaluating the effect of colesvelam hydrochloride on glycemic control in subjects with type 2 diabetes. *Clin Ther* 29:74–83, 2007

16. Fonseca VA, Rosenstock J, Wang AC, Truitt KE, Jones MR: Colesevelam HCl improves glycemic control and reduces LDL cholesterol in patients with inadequately controlled type 2 diabetes on sulfonylurea-based therapy. *Diabetes Care* 31:1479–1484, 2008

Chapter 5
Hypertension

BACKGROUND

The beneficial effects of lowering blood pressure on cardiovascular disease are well substantiated in Chapter 1. Because the risk for clinical cardiovascular disease events (heart attacks and strokes) and cardiovascular disease mortality is much higher in people with diabetes, the benefit in people with diabetes is greater in this population than in a population without diabetes. The beneficial effects of lowering blood pressure on microvascular complications were also mentioned in Chapter 1 but not described in detail. Figure 5 shows the critical importance of achieving the American Diabetes Association systolic blood pressure goal of <130 mmHg on forestalling deterioration of kidney function.

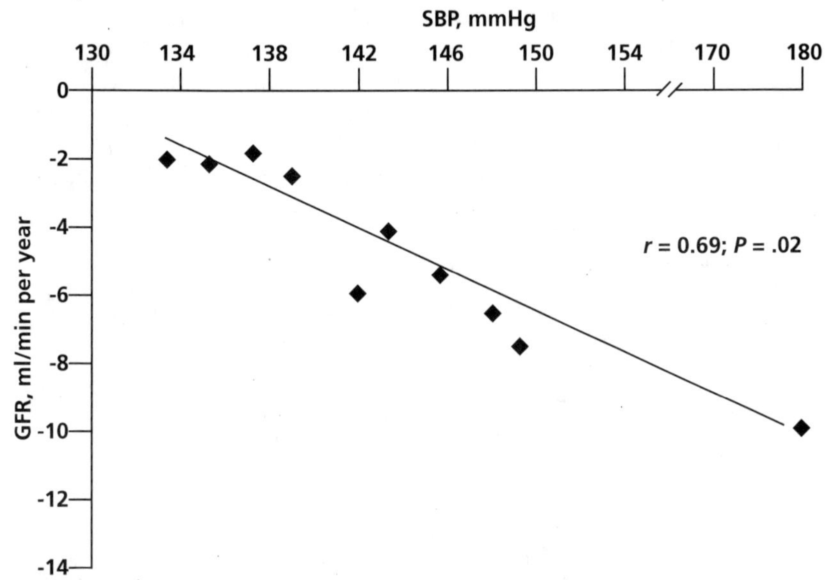

Figure 5. Rates of decline in glomerular filtration rate (GFR) versus systolic blood pressure (SBP) in studies extending for ≥3 years in patients with type 2 diabetes nephropathy. Adapted from Reference 4.

There are 10 classes of antihypertensive drugs but no class is clearly more effective than any other in lowering blood pressure. Therefore, decisions about which class(es) to use revolve around any other additional benefits independent of their effect on blood pressure. As described in Chapter 1, angiotensin converting enzyme (ACE) inhibitors and angiotensin receptor blockers (ARBs) reduce microalbuminuria and clinical proteinuria independent of their blood pressure–lowering effect. There is no significant difference in cardiovascular disease outcomes among the different classes of drugs, their benefits being related to the extent of blood pressure lowering (1). Some recommend abandoning the stepped-care approach to treating hypertension (where one drug is increased to its maximum dose before adding another one) and initiating treatment with a combination of two drugs at submaximal doses (2). This approach is based on two factors: *1*) increasing doses in the upper part of the dose-response range gives less effect of that in the lower part; and *2*) the majority of diabetic patients will require more than one drug to meet the blood pressure goal. However, these algorithms to treat hypertension retain the stepped-care approach for four reasons: *1*) to limit exposure to the side effects of different classes of drugs unless necessary, i.e., when the goal is not met with maximum doses of drug(s) in the class(es) used; *2*) evaluation of the effect of increasing the dose of a drug or introducing a new class takes place in 1 month, so that rapid titration of drugs to achieve the goal occurs, and patients are not exposed to elevated blood pressure levels for long periods of time; *3*) the maximal dose of a single drug is just as effective as submaximal doses of two drugs (3); and *4*) progressive increases of submaximal doses of more than one drug is more difficult algorithmically.

Each class of antihypertensive drugs (in alphabetical order) is briefly described, and the individual drugs are listed in Table 16. A simplified version of the renin-angiotensin system is provided in Figure 6 to aid in understanding the mechanisms of action of the four classes of drugs that affect these pathways.

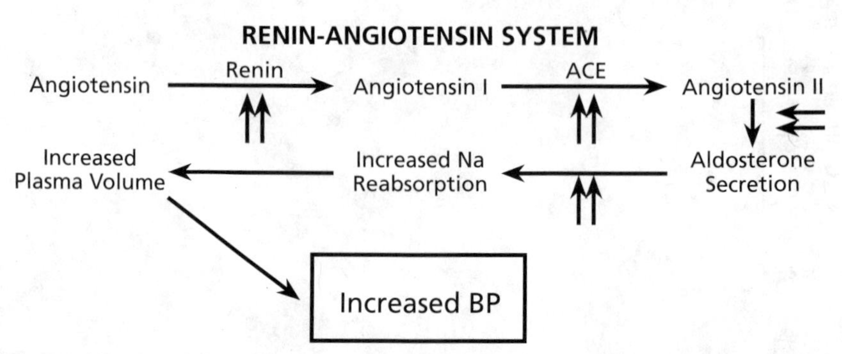

Figure 6. Simplified version of the renin-angiotensin system. Double arrows denote sites of inhibition of antihypertensive drugs. See text for discussion.

Table 16. Antihypertensive Oral Medications

Generic Name	Brand Name	Dosage Size Availability
ACE Inhibitor		
Benazepril	Lotensin, generic	5, 10, 20, 40 mg tablet
Captopril	Capoten, generic	12.5, 25, 50, 100 mg tablet
Enalapril	Vasotec, generic	2.5, 5, 10, 20 mg tablet
Fosinopril	Monopril, generic	10, 20, 40 mg tablet
Lisinopril	Prinivil, Zestril, generic	2.5, 5, 10, 20, 30, 40 mg tablet
Moexipril	Univasc, generic	7.5, 15 mg tablet
Perindopril	Aceon	2, 4, 8 mg tablet
Quinapril	Accupril, generic	5, 10, 20, 40 mg tablet
Ramipril	Altace, generic	1.25, 2.5, 5, 10 mg tablet
Trandolapril	Mavik, generic	1, 2, 4 mg tablet
Angiotensin II Receptor Antagonist (ARB)		
Candesartan	Atacand	4, 8, 16, 32 mg tablet
Eprosartan	Tevetan	400, 600 mg tablet
Irbesartan	Avapro	75, 150, 300 mg tablet
Losartan	Cozaar	25, 50, 100 mg tablet
Olmesartan	Benacar	5, 20, 40 mg tablet
Telmisartan	Micardis	20, 40, 80 mg tablet
Valsartan	Diovan, generic	40, 80, 160, 320 mg tablet
Calcium Channel Blocker		
Amlodipine	Norvasc, generic	2.5, 5, 10 mg tablet
Diltiazem	Cardizem, generic Cardizem CD, generic Cardizem LA, generic Cardizem SR, generic	30, 60, 90 mg tablet 120, 180, 240, 300 mg capsule 120, 240, 360, 420 mg tablet 120 mg capsule
Felodipine	Plendil, generic	2.5, 5, 10 mg tablet
Isradipine	Dynacirc, generic Dynacirc Cr, generic	2.5, 5 mg tablet 5 mg tablet
Nifedipine	Procardia, generic Procardia XL, generic	10 mg capsule 30, 60, 90 mg capsule

Generic Name	Brand Name	Dosage Size Availability
Nicardipne	Cardene, generic Cardene SR, generic	20, 30 mg capsule 30, 45, 60 mg capsule
Nisoldipine	Sular, generic	8.5, 17, 25.5, 34 mg tablet
Verapamil	Calan, generic Calan SR, generic	40, 80, 160 mg tablet 120, 180, 240 mg tablet
Renin Inhibitor		
Aliskiren	Tekturna	150, 300 mg tablet
Aldosterone Receptor Antagonist (Blocker)		
Eplerenone	Inspra	25, 50 mg tablet
Spironolactone	Aldactone, generic	25, 50, 100 mg tablet
β-Adrenergic Blocker		
Acebutolol	Sectral, generic	200, 400 mg capsule
Atenolol	Tenormin, generic	25, 50, 100 mg tablet
Betaxolol	Kerlone, generic	10, 20 mg tablet
Bisoprolol	Zebeta, generic	5, 10 mg tablet
Carteolol	Cartrol, generic	2.5, 5 mg tablet
Carvedilol	Coreg, generic	3.125, 6.25, 12.5, 25 mg tablet
Labetalol	Trandate, generic	100, 200, 300 mg tablet
Metoprolol	Lopressor, generic Toprol XL, generic	50, 100 mg tablet 25, 50, 100, 200 mg tablet
Naldolol	Corgard, generic	20, 40, 80, 160 mg tablet
Nebivolol	Bystolic	2.5, 5, 10, 20 mg tablet
Penbutolol	Levatol	20 mg tablet
Pindolol	Visken, generic	5, 10 mg tablet
Propanolol	Inderal, generic Inderal LA, generic	10, 20, 40, 60, 80 mg tablet 60, 80, 120, 160 mg tablet
Timolol	Blocadren, generic	5, 10, 20 mg tablet
α-Adrenergic Receptor Antagonist (Blocker)		
Doxazosin	Cardura, generic Cardura XL, generic	1, 2, 4, 8 mg tablet 4, 8 mg tablet
Prazosin	Minipress, generic	1, 2, 5 mg capsule
Terazosin	Hytrin, generic	1, 2, 5, 10 mg capsule

Generic Name	Brand Name	Dosage Size Availability
Vasodilator		
Hydralazine	Apresoline, generic	10, 25, 50, 100 mg tablet
Minoxidil	Loniten, generic	2.5, 10 mg tablet
α-Adrenergic Agonist (Sympatholytics)		
Clonidine	Catapres, generic	0.1, 0.2, 0.3 mg tablet
Guanabenz	Wytensin, generic	4, 8 mg tablet
Methyldopa	Aldomet, generic	250, 500 mg tablet
Reserpine	Serpalan, generic Serpasil, generic	0.1, 0.25 mg tablet
Loop Diuretic		
Bumetanide	Bumex, generic	0.5, 1, 2 mg tablet
Ethacrynic acid	Edecrin, generic	25 mg tablet
Furosemide	Lasix, generic	20, 40, 80 mg tablet
Torsemide	Demadex, generic	10, 20 mg tablet
Potassium Sparing Diuretic		
Amiloride	Midamor, generic	5 mg tablet
Triamterene	Dyrenium, generic	50, 100 mg tablet
Thiazide Diuretic		
Chlorothiazide	Diuril, generic	250, 500 mg tablet; 250 mg/5-ml suspension
Chlorthalidone	Thalitone, generic	15, 25, 50, 100 mg tablet
Hydrochloro-thiazide	HydroDIURIL, generic	25, 50 mg tablet; 12.5 mg capsule
Methychloro-thiazide	Aquatensen, generic	5 mg tablet
Polythiazide	Renese, generic	1, 2 mg tablet
Indapamide	Lozol, generic	1.25, 2.5 mg tablet
Metolozone	Zaroxolyn, generic	2.5, 5, 10 mg tablet

ALDOSTERONE RECEPTOR ANTAGONISTS (BLOCKERS)

Aldosterone acts on the distal tubule and collecting ducts in the kidney to promote sodium reabsorption and potassium excretion. Enhanced sodium reabsorption increases plasma volume, which contributes to hypertension. Aldosterone blockers lead to enhanced sodium excretion and potassium retention. The former decreases the increased plasma volume associated with hypertension and is the major basis of their antihypertensive effect. The latter is the basis of one of their potential side effects, hyperkalemia. The nonselective aldosterone blocker, spironolactone, also binds to the progesterone and androgen receptors, which can cause the side effects of menstrual abnormalities in premenopausal women and gynecomastia, breast pain, and impotence in men. Eplerenone, a selective aldosterone blocker, binds only weakly to the progesterone and androgen receptors and does not cause these side effects.

α_1-ADRENERGIC RECEPTOR ANTAGONISTS (BLOCKERS)

α_1-Adrenergic receptors are located predominantly post-synaptically on vascular smooth muscle cells, where they are the principal sites of the vasoconstrictive action of norepinephrine. Because sympathetic overactivity is associated with hypertension, blocking these receptors is the basis of their anti-hypertensive effect. Side effects are minimal with the exception of the "first-dose phenomenon," which is severe orthostatic (postural) hypotension with initial exposure to the drug. This initial effect usually disappears rapidly after further doses, presumably because of subsequent salt and water retention (although occasionally mild postural hypotension may persist). To avoid this negative clinical effect, it is recommended that the first dose be 1.0 mg to be taken at bedtime, so that the patient will not be exposed to orthostasis. The first-dose phenomenon can also occur if the α_1-receptor antagonists are added to other antihypertensive medications. Since α_1-adrenergic receptors also regulate the degree of constriction of urinary tract sphincters (they are commonly used to treat benign prostatic hypertrophy), individuals with alterations of urinary bladder function may experience incontinence with α_1-receptor blockade due to relaxation of the bladder outlet.

α_2-ADRENERGIC RECEPTOR AGONISTS (CENTRAL AND PERIPHERAL SYMPATHOLYTICS)

α_2-Adrenergic receptors are located pre-synaptically in the central nervous system and post-synaptically in the peripheral nervous system. When they are activated in the brain by centrally acting drugs, sympathetic outflow to the heart and blood vessels is inhibited. This diminution of sympathetic tone reduces cardiac output and peripheral vascular resistance, thereby lowering blood pressure. They should be used with caution with β-blockers because of their synergistic effects to induce bradycardia. The most common adverse effects of central sympatholytics are dry mouth and somnolence (up to 40% of patients). Hypersensitivity reactions with methyldopa, commonly used to treat hypertension in pregnancy, may occur, including hepatitis and a Coombs-positive hemolytic anemia. Rebound hypertension may occur if clonidine is discontinued abruptly, especially if higher doses (≥1.0 mg) are being used. Skin hypersensitivity to the clonidine patch is not uncommon (up to 20% of patients).

Peripheral sympatholytics deplete norepinephrine from the post-ganglionic sympathetic nerves, which reduces cardiac and neurogenic vascular tone. This decreases cardiac output and peripheral vascular resistance, thereby lowering blood pressure. Reserpine, which also works centrally, commonly causes nasal stuffiness and has been associated with significant depression. Other adverse effects of these drugs include orthostatic hypotension, retrograde ejaculation, increased gastric acidity, and risk of acid-peptic disease as well as increased intestinal motility leading to increased stools. A hypertensive crisis may be precipitated if these drugs are used with monoamine oxidase inhibitors.

ACE INHIBITORS

The role of aldosterone in the pathogenesis of hypertension and the effect of blocking its actions in treatment are described under Aldosterone Receptor Antagonists (Blocker) above. The effect of ACE inhibitors in treating hypertension is mainly due to decreasing aldosterone secretion. Angiotensin I is converted by ACE to angiotensin II, which then binds to the angiotensin II receptor and stimulates the release of aldosterone. An ACE inhibitor blocks this conversion, which lowers angiotensin II and therefore its subsequent stimulation of the release of aldosterone.

The two major side effects of ACE inhibitors are hyperkalemia, which is more likely to occur in patients with renal insufficiency, and a dry, nonproductive cough in ~10% of patients. This occurs because the ACE also breaks down bradykinin, which accumulates in the presence of ACE inhibitors and causes the cough. The cough typically disappears 1–2 weeks after discontinuing the ACE inhibitor. A rare, but potentially life-threatening, side effect occurring in <1% of patients is angioneurotic edema. If this should occur, the patient can be switched to an ARB, since angioedema is much less common with this class of drugs. ACE inhibitors are contraindicated in pregnancy because of their effect on the fetus manifested in the second and third trimesters.

Because there is a wide variation in the responses of African Americans to ACE inhibitors, it is incorrectly believed that these patients do not respond as well to this class of drugs as other populations. If doses are adequately titrated, most patients will respond. Racial differences are abolished when a thiazide diuretic (see below) is added to an ACE inhibitor. ACE inhibitor therapy in patients with renal artery stenosis can produce renal insufficiency. ACE inhibitors are also indicated in patients with heart failure and after a myocardial infarction, independent of their effects on blood pressure.

ANGIOTENSIN RECEPTOR ANTAGONISTS (BLOCKERS)

ARBs block the binding of angiotensin to its receptor, thereby decreasing aldosterone secretion. As with the ACE inhibitors, early studies suggested that African Americans may not respond as well, although later studies showed good responses to higher doses. Racial differences also disappear when ARBs are combined with a thiazide diuretic. Cough and angioneurotic edema are not increased in patients taking ARBs, although, as expected, hyperkalemia is. A few of the patients who experienced angioneurotic edema on ACE inhibitor treatment may also have it when switched to an ARB, but usually not. As with ACE inhibitors, ARBs are also contraindicated in pregnancy.

β-ADRENERGIC RECEPTOR ANTAGONISTS (BLOCKERS)

Even though β-blockers have been used for many years to control hypertension, their mechanism is still not clear. It probably involves many systems, such as *1*) reducing heart rate and cardiac output; *2*) central nervous system effects; *3*) inhibition of renin release (renin catalyzes the formation of angiotensin I from its precursor, angiotensinogen); and *4*) dilating the peripheral vessels. Other systems may be involved as well. β-Blockers are classically divided into lipid- and water-soluble compounds. The lipid-soluble drugs are eliminated largely by hepatic metabolism, have shorter half-lives, and have more variable plasma concentrations. Water-soluble drugs are eliminated unchanged by the kidneys, have longer half-lives, and have more stable plasma concentrations. Because they are eliminated by the kidneys, water-soluble β-blockers (e.g., atenolol) should be used with caution in patients with marked renal insufficiency. However, β-blockers have similar antihypertensive effects despite these pharmacokinetic differences.

There are several other differences among β-blockers, one of which involves their effects on different β-adrenergic receptors. From a clinical perspective, the two important β-adrenergic receptors are β_1-receptors, which are located in the heart, and β_2-receptors, which are located on the pulmonary bronchi. Activation of β_1-receptors increases cardiac output and heart rate so that inhibition of these effects by β_1-adrenergic blockers (termed cardioselective drugs) would lower blood pressure. Activation of β_2-receptors dilates the bronchi (the basis of inhaled β_2-receptor agonist treatment for asthma) so that inhibition of this effect by a nonselective β-blocker (i.e., a drug that blocks both β_1- and β_2-adrenergic receptors) could exacerbate pulmonary disease. In higher doses, however, β_1-selective blocking agents also block β_2 receptors.

Two β-adrenergic blockers (carvediol and labetalol) also block α-adrenergic receptors. Although they are useful in the treatment of hypertension (and angina pectoris), the additional effect on the α-receptors reduces peripheral vascular resistance, which can lead to higher cardiac output.

Several β-blockers (acebutol, carteolol, penbutolol, pindolol, and possibly labetalol) are also partial agonists, i.e., they initially stimulate the receptor before blocking it. This intrinsic sympathomimetic activity does not reduce resting heart rate (as opposed to other β-blockers) but does blunt the increased heart rate during exercise when the sympathetic nervous system is stimulated. These agents are just as effective in treating hypertension as agents without intrinsic sympathomimetic activity.

β-Blockers without intrinsic sympathomimetic activity reduce resting heart rates, and most physicians will not increase the dose if the pulse is <70 beats per minute. In patients with coronary heart disease, abrupt discontinuation of a β-blocker, especially if given in high doses, can precipitate angina and therefore should be tapered slowly. In general, β-blockers should not be used in patients with asthma, chronic obstructive pulmonary disease, heart block greater than first degree, and sick sinus syndrome. Although it is commonly stated that β-blockers should not be used in insulin-requiring patients because they may blunt the symptoms of, and possibly the recovery from, hypoglycemia, this has not been much of a clinical problem. β-Blockers should be used with caution with the non-dihydropyridine calcium channel blockers, verapamil and diltiazem, because the combination further depresses the sinoatrial and atrioventricular nodes, with the latter leading to a possible atrioventricular block.

CALCIUM CHANNEL ANTAGONISTS (BLOCKERS)

There are several subtypes of calcium channels, but the L-type channel is the one most directly associated with blood pressure. Calcium channel blockers block these channels resulting in arteriolar dilatation, which reduces peripheral vascular resistance and results in lowered blood pressure levels. There are two broad classes of calcium channel blockers: non-dihydropyridines (verapamil and diltiazem) and dihydropyridines (which include the rest). Withdrawal of calcium channel blockers does not cause rebound hypertension, but rapid withdrawal may induce coronary spasm and angina pectoris, especially in patients with ischemic heart disease. Calcium channel blockers are generally well tolerated. Their side effects are related to their effect as arteriolar dilators and include headache, flushing, tachycardia (especially the dihydropyridines), and edema. The non-dihydropyridines are less likely to cause edema. As stated above, because of their effect on depressing the sinoatrial and atrioventricular nodes, non-dihydropyridines can decrease the heart rate and should be used with caution with β-blockers.

RENIN INHIBITORS

Renin, secreted by the kidney, converts angiotensinogen, secreted mainly by the liver, to angiotensin I (which is the precursor of angiotensin II, which stimulates the release of aldosterone). Therefore, inhibitors of renin release lower blood pressure by interfering at an early step in the renin-angiotensin system.

Currently, aliskiren is the only approved drug in this class. Occasional adverse effects include rare angioedema, hyperkalemia (especially when used with ACE inhibitors), hypotension (particularly in volume-depleted patients), diarrhea and other gastrointestinal symptoms, rash, and mildly elevated uric acid levels. No clinically important interactions with other drugs have been reported.

THIAZIDES AND LOOP DIURETICS

Because expansion of the extracellular fluid volume characterizes the hypertension in people with diabetes, thiazide diuretics are an excellent choice. They act by inhibiting the reabsorption of sodium from the collecting tubules in the kidney back into the bloodstream, thus increasing urinary sodium excretion and initially reducing the extracellular fluid volume. However, this initial volume contraction does not persist and reverses within a few days. Chronically, a vasodilation effect of thiazide diuretics (by unclear mechanisms) reduces peripheral vascular resistance and controls blood pressure by this means.

Thiazide diuretics do not work well in the presence of renal insufficiency and should not be used if the estimated glomerular filtration rate (eGFR) is <50 ml/min or, if this value is not available, if the serum creatinine level is ≥1.9 mg/dl.

Clinically significant adverse effects of thiazide diuretics are few. Potassium loss occurs mostly within the first week of therapy, and overall reductions in serum potassium levels are usually ≤0.3 mEq/l. If hypokalemia is a problem, a potassium-sparing diuretic (or potassium supplements) can be used. Fewer than 10% of patients on 12.5 or 25 mg daily of hydrochlorothiazide may develop mild hypokalemia, but since ACE inhibitors or ARBs are usually also being taken by diabetic patients, hypokalemia is even less of a problem. Thiazide diuretics may also cause slight increases in uric acid and decreases in magnesium levels, but these rarely are of clinical significance. An occasional patient may have hyponatremia, especially in individuals who become dehydrated. Because thiazides contain sulfur, they should not be used in the rare patient who is allergic to sulfur.

Loop diuretics also inhibit sodium reabsorption from the kidney back into the bloodstream, but at a different site from thiazide diuretics. They are often used in patients with renal insufficiency and in those with edema. In patients with normal renal function, the initial increase in sodium excretion is often followed by rebound sodium retention. Because they do not affect peripheral vascular resistance, blood pressure may not be consistently reduced, especially if loop diuretics are taken only once a day. (With the exception of toresamide, loop diuretics are short-acting.) In general, the adverse effects of the loop diuretics are similar to thiazide diuretics, except they may increase urinary calcium loss, which usually is also not a clinical problem.

VASODILATORS (DIRECT)

These arterial dilator drugs act directly on vascular smooth muscle cells, causing relaxation and vasodilation, which decreases peripheral vascular resistance and thereby lowers blood pressure. If used as monotherapy, patients rapidly develop tolerance to them as a result of reflex increases in sympathetic nervous system activity, activation of the rennin-angiotensin system (described above), and sodium retention. They should be used in combination with antiadrenergic drugs (a β-blocker or a central sympatholytic), diuretics, and/or ACE inhibitors or ARBs. As used in the algorithms presented below, they are a fourth-line drug.

Inactivation of hydralazine by acetylation is genetically determined, with about half of the U.S. population being "slow" acetylators. These individuals (who have a higher plasma concentration after an oral dose than "fast" acetylators) are more likely to have adverse effects. These include nausea and vomiting, occasionally peripheral neuropathy, and, at higher doses (>200 mg/day) in slow acetylators, a lupus-like syndrome more commonly in women, appearing 6–24 months after starting the drug. But this condition is rapidly reversible when the drug is stopped. In cases where hydralazine-induced lupus is suspected, note that antibodies, often in high titers, are to single-stranded DNA as opposed to the native double-stranded DNA seen in women with classic lupus erythematosis.

Minoxidil, an extremely effective vasodilator, has similar overall hemodynamic actions to hydralazine. It does not have the adverse effect of a lupus-like syndrome but does cause (reversible) hair growth, which limits its use in women. The drug is usually used only in patients whose blood pressure is refractory to the combination of many other classes of drugs.

HYPERTENSION ALGORITHM

Drug choices are limited to those available in the Los Angeles County formulary.

TREATMENT PLAN

1. Initial hypertension treatment for blood pressure <160/100 mmHg is medical nutritional therapy (MNT) and lifestyle modification.
2. Pharmacologic therapy is initiated on any patient who does not meet the goal of ≤130/80 mmHg and has failed MNT and lifestyle modification for ~4–8 weeks.
3. Principles of treatment to achieve the blood pressure goal of ≤130/80 mmHg:
   a) To determine the effect of starting or changing the dose of an anti-hypertensive medication, measure the blood pressure ~4 weeks after initiating or changing the dose.
   b) If blood pressure goal of ≤130/80 mmHg is not reached at the maximal (tolerated) dose of a class of drugs, add the drug from the next class.

A. Non-pharmacologic therapy (lifestyle change)

- Weight reduction toward desirable body weight of at least 5–10% of initial weight
- Salt restriction to as close to 2 g/day as possible, using the DASH (Dietary Approaches to Stop Hypertension) diet
- Smoking cessation
- Limit daily alcohol intake to <2 oz/day
- Exercise (walking, swimming, etc., 30–45 min 3–4 times per week)
- Caffeine cessation
- Stress reduction
- If blood pressure is controlled at ≤130/80 mmHg, continue with non-pharmacologic program
- Lifestyle modification for 8 weeks. If blood pressure goal of ≤130/80 mmHg is not met, go to B.

B. First-line drug(s) for pharmacologic treatment (ACE inhibitors or ARBs)

1. Start patient on 10 mg benazepril (an ACE inhibitor) once daily.
2. Measure K^+ 2 weeks after each change of benazepril dose.
3. If K^+ is above the upper limit of normal, decrease to previous dose.

4. Increase benazepril to 20 mg once daily if blood pressure goal not met at 4-week follow-up.
5. Measure K^+ 2 weeks after dose increase; if above the upper limit of normal, decrease to previous dose.
6. Increase benazepril to 40 mg once daily (maximal anti-hypertension dose) if blood pressure goal not met at 4-week follow-up.
7. Measure K^+ 2 weeks after dose increase; if above the upper limit of normal, decrease to previous dose.
8. If patient complains of a cough or angioneurotic edema (two other side effects in addition to hyperkalemia), discontinue benazepril and start losartan (Cozaar), an ARB using a dose equivalency from Table 17.
9. Because ARBs also raise K^+ levels, they cannot be substituted for an ACE inhibitor if the latter causes hyperkalemia.
10. If the blood pressure goal of ≤130/80 mmHg is not met at the 4-week follow-up visit after the maximal dose of an ACE inhibitor or an ARB is prescribed, go to C.

Table 17. Dose Equivalency

ACE inhibitor	ARB
Benazepril 10 mg	Losartan 20 mg
Benazepril 20 mg	Losartan 50 mg
Benazepril 40 mg	Losartan 100 mg

C. Second-line drug (diuretic): Hydrochlorothiazide (if eGFR is ≥50 ml/min [or if unavailable, serum creatinine is ≤1.8 mg/dl]) or indapamide (Lozol) (if eGFR is <50 ml/min [or if unavailable, serum creatinine is ≥1.9 mg/dl], see #4 below). To be used if blood pressure goal of ≤130/80 is not achieved with a maximal (tolerated) dose of an ACE inhibitor or ARB.

1. Add 12.5 mg hydrochlorothiazide once daily.
2. If blood pressure goal of ≤130/80 mmHg is not met at the 4-week follow-up visit, increase hydrochlorothiazide to 25 mg once daily (maximal dose).
3. If blood pressure goal of ≤130/80 mmHg is not met at the 4-week follow-up visit, go to D.
4. If the eGFR is <50 ml/min (or if unavailable, serum creatinine is ≥1.9 mg/dl), start indapamide 1.25 mg once daily.
5. If blood pressure goal of ≤130/80 mmHg is not met at the 4-week

follow-up visit, increase indapamide dose to 2.5 mg once daily (maximal dose).
6. If blood pressure goal of ≤130/80 mmHg is not met at the 4-week follow-up visit, go to D.

D. Third-line drug (non-dihydropyridine calcium channel blocker): Diltiazem (Cardiazem) or verapamil (Calan). To be used if blood pressure goal of ≤130/80 mmHg is not achieved with combination of maximal doses of the first- and second-line drugs.
1. Add 180 mg diltiazem ER (or verapamil ER) once daily.
2. If the blood pressure goal of ≤130/80 mmHg is not met at the 4-week follow-up visit, increase to 180 mg twice daily (maximal dose).
3. If blood pressure goal of ≤130/80 mmHg is not met at the 4-week follow-up visit and the patient is at the maximum dose of a combination of the first-, second-, and third-line drugs, go to E.

E. Fourth-line drug (direct vasodilators) (hydralazine): To be used if blood pressure goal of ≤130/80 mmHg is not achieved with a combination of maximal doses of first-, second-, and third-line drugs.
1. Add 50 mg hydralazine twice daily.
2. If blood pressure goal of ≤130/80 mmHg is not met at 4-week follow-up visit, increase to 100 mg twice daily (maximal dose).
3. If blood pressure goal of ≤130/80 mmHg is not met at 4-week follow-up visit and patient is taking maximal doses of four classes of drugs (ACE inhibitor or ARB, diuretic, non-dihydropyridine calcium channel blocker, and direct vasodilator), CONSULT MD.

References

1. Blood Pressure Lowering Treatment Collaboration: Effects of different blood-pressure regimens on major cardiovascular events: results of prospectively-designed overviews of randomized trials. *Lancet* 362:1527–1535, 2003

2. Wald DS, Law M, Morris JK, Bestwick JP, Wald NJ: Combination therapy versus monotherapy in reducing blood pressure: meta-analysis on 11,000 participants from 42 trials. *Am J Med* 122:290–300, 2009

3. Anderson NH, Poulsen PL, Knudsen ST, Poulsen SH, Eiskjer H, Hansen KW, Helleberg K, Mogensen CE: Long-term dual blockade with candesartan and lisinopril in hypertensive patients with diabetes: the CALM II study. *Diabetes Care* 28:273–277, 2005

4. Bakris GJ: A practical approach to achieving recommended blood pressure goals in diabetic patients. *Arch Intern Med* 161:2661–2667, 2001

Index

B

C

H

I

J

K

L

M

Q

R

S

T

U

V

W

Z